You brush your t[eeth]... teeth clean. You [...] to supplement yo[...] multiple times per day to keep your job. What is your daily practice to strengthen the integration of your mind, body, and spirit? Think of *Designed to Heal* by Dr. Ben Rall as your daily spiritual dose for health and wholeness.

—KEVIN W. MCCARTHY
AUTHOR, *THE ON-PURPOSE PERSON*

What a simple yet transformative book! Easy to read and use in daily life, this book has the ability to completely transform your health and life in a short amount of time per day without more prescriptions or doctor visits and honoring the way God created the world and designed our bodies.

—DAN SULLIVAN, DC
AUTHOR, *THE TRUST FORMULA*

I read Dr. Rall's *Cooperative Wellness* book several years ago and was amazed at how he simplified how you can take control of your health instead of relying on the broken healthcare system that plagues our country today. I've been able to use that knowledge to help my clients and even to teach my own kids how they can live differently and honor the power God put in their bodies to heal. I'm not at all surprised that Dr. Ben's latest book, *Designed to Heal*, is just as powerful as his first! He makes living a faithful and healthy lifestyle simple by combining some of the most influential and powerful passages of Scripture with doable action steps that can lead to a renewing of mind, body, and spirit.

—DANIEL HUCK, MS, CPT, CFNC
ENTREPRENEUR AND MEN'S WELLNESS COACH

Dr. Ben Rall has done a remarkable job integrating a biblical worldview into his practice and care for his patients. He understands how God has designed the body to work and how to help fix many health problems our modern medical industry wants to simply medicate without getting to the root of the problem. His meditations on Scripture and our health will prove helpful in enabling us to be mindful of the amazing bodies God has given us to steward. He is a trusted voice in my and my family's healthcare.

—ROSS MIDDLETON
ASSOCIATE PASTOR, HIGHPOINT CHURCH ORLANDO

God calls us to be bold and courageous and not conform to this world. So many Christians are complacent in the face of evil and act like the Israelites, who fled in fear when they saw Goliath. This book helps you put your faith into action, be like David, and tackle whatever giants you might be facing.

—BEN TAPPER, DC
PRODUCER, *THE TIME IS NOW*

Dr. Rall's book is a rare find in the transformation genre. His daily inspirations truly focus on wholeness for body, soul, and spirit. In today's world, our quick-fix mentality usually fails to acknowledge the totality of who we are. This is a refreshing and well-written book that gives readers tangible action steps that address their whole being.

—MATT TONNOS, DC
COFOUNDER, THE CHIROPRACTIC REVOLUTION

Dr. Ben ties physical health to spiritual health using strong passages of Scripture. He exhorts us to take action to care for ourselves in body, soul, and mind. *Designed to Heal* is a daily inspiration for doctors, patients, and Christ-followers. The short devotionals are power-packed. They challenge readers to reflect and take a personal account for where they are and to repent if necessary.

—DAVID K. ERB, DC
COAUTHOR, *BREAKING FREE FROM CHEMICAL RELIGION*

I have been both blessed and challenged by Dr. Ben's unrelenting passion to disciple others toward the truth that their bodies truly are amazing creations with a design for healing. These words in this book will challenge conventional wisdom and open your eyes to what your Creator has to say about what is really wise.

—JEFF MCLAUGHLIN
PRODUCER AND COHOST, *DESIGNED TO HEAL* PODCAST

It is essential for every person to understand the importance of being healthy and whole in mind, body, and spirit. In his book *Designed to Heal*, Dr. Ben Rall masterfully outlines a day-by-day blueprint for those who desire to grow in these areas of their lives by sharing his vast knowledge, life experience, and wisdom on these topics. This book is specifically designed to challenge you to grow in faith, take action, and achieve your goals. It has worked for me. Now get ready for it to work for you!

—ROBERT J. ENGE III
EXECUTIVE ASSISTANT, CHRIST FOR ALL NATIONS

Designed to Heal is a powerful tool for renewing your mind and being intentional on your journey to live a life of health and impact. In order for us to thrive in this day and age, we have to establish the habit of quiet time, reading, and contemplation. This book from Dr. Ben Rall is an incredible resource that will bless you and challenge you toward your highest level of health and contribution.

—TERRY HARMON, DC
FOUNDER, C.A.M.P. LIFESTYLE ACADEMY

Dr. Ben Rall has been a consistent blessing to me and my family. We became friends over the topic of money and faith, but grew closer as he began providing life-giving care to my whole family. He isn't afraid of hard work or hard truth, and through these short, powerful daily reflections he encourages us to embrace the life-giving message of the Bible.

—JOHN CORTINES
COAUTHOR, *GOD AND MONEY AND TRUE RICHES*

There is a great grace throughout the pages of *Designed to Heal* to go deeper with God. You will be inspired by the daily encouragement as you learn the unforced rhythms of God's grace to contend for the miraculous and live a more prudent life by gaining wisdom in the practical matters of life and health.

—PETE SULACK, DC
FOUNDER, MATTHEW 10 INTERNATIONAL

Dr. Ben provides a simple, Scripture-based devotional that provides a quick but convicting thought for the day. It is not filled with fluff or emotions but shoots straight to the heart of the gospel and inspires the reader to look closely at his or her role in being whole and healthy for the kingdom.

—JODI MOCKABEE
BEST-SELLING AUTHOR, *THE WHOLE AND HEALTHY FAMILY*

designed to heal

BEN RALL, DC

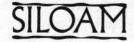

DESIGNED TO HEAL by Ben Rall, DC
Published by Siloam, an imprint of Charisma Media
600 Rinehart Road, Lake Mary, Florida 32746

For more Spirit-led resources, visit charismahouse.com and
the author's website at achievewellness.clinic.

Cataloging-in-Publication Data is on file with the Library of Congress.

International Standard Book Number: 978-1-63641-239-9

E-book ISBN: 978-1-63641-240-5

23 24 25 26 27 — 987654321

Printed in the United States of America

Most Charisma Media products are available at special quantity discounts for bulk purchase for sales promotions, premiums, fund-raising, and educational needs. For details, call us at (407) 333-0600 or visit our website at www. charismamedia.com.

This book contains the opinions and ideas of its author. It is solely for informational and educational purposes and should not be regarded as a substitute for professional medical treatment. The nature of your body's health condition is complex and unique. Therefore, you should consult a health professional before you begin any new exercise, nutrition, or supplementation program or if you have questions about your health. Neither the author nor the publisher shall be liable or responsible for any loss or damage allegedly arising from any information or suggestion in this book.

The statements in this book about consumable products or food have not been evaluated by the Food and Drug Administration. The recipes in this book are to be followed exactly as written. The publisher is not responsible for your specific health or allergy needs that may require medical supervision. The publisher is not responsible for any adverse reactions to the consumption of food or products that have been suggested in this book.

This book is dedicated to all the patients I have been honored to serve, and to my favorite patients—my wife, Megan, and children, Grace and Jack.

CONTENTS

Preface xxi

Introduction xxii

Day 1   In the Beginning, God 1

Day 2   Divine Design. 2

Day 3   He Is a God of More Than Enough!. 3

Day 4   Sabbath 4

Day 5   He Is the Breath in Our Lungs 5

Day 6   Work It...With Others 6

Day 7   What Did He Say? Did He Really Say That? 7

Day 8   120 8

Day 9   The Rainbow 9

Day 10   Are You Willing? 10

Day 11   Grumbling in the Desert 11

Day 12   Sometimes We Need to Follow the Recipe 12

Day 13   American Idol 13

Day 14   Are You Radiating? 14

Day 15   Do Not... 15

Day 16   Where Did Everybody Go? 16

Day 17   Blessed for Obedience. 17

Day 18   Digest the Word of God. 18

Day 19   He Will Never Leave or Forsake You 19

Day 20   And the Walls Came Down! 20

Day 21   Prayers That Stop Time 21

Day 22   Don't Tell Me What to Do 22

Day 23   Be an Influencer 23

Day 24   What Goes On Goes In. 24

Day 25   What Is Your Anointing?. 25

Day 26   What's Your Goliath? 26

Day 27   But I Really Messed Up 27

Day 28   Resurrected 28

Day 29	God of Miracles...and Miracles...and Miracles	29
Day 30	Pride	30
Day 31	Do You Have a Heart Condition?	31
Day 32	Fire From Heaven	32
Day 33	The Naysayers	33
Day 34	No Excuses	34
Day 35	For a Time Such as This	35
Day 36	Will You Pass the Test?	36
Day 37	All for Nothing	37
Day 38	When Friends Fail	38
Day 39	Perverted	39
Day 40	Where Were You When I Created It All?	40
Day 41	Water Your Plants!	41
Day 42	Who Is Your Shepherd?	42
Day 43	Create in Me a Clean Heart, O Lord!	43
Day 44	Bones Heal	44
Day 45	The Heart of the Matter	45
Day 46	They Are Corrupt	46
Day 47	When Your Flesh Fails	47
Day 48	A Blameless Walk	48
Day 49	This Is Your Brain on Sugar	49
Day 50	Are You Thankful?	50
Day 51	The Lord's Protection	51
Day 52	Each of Us Is Unique	52
Day 53	He Knows Each of Us by Name	53
Day 54	He Hung the Moon!	54
Day 55	Make Time	55
Day 56	Trust the Lord	56
Day 57	Are You Wise?	57
Day 58	Discipline Is Freedom	58
Day 59	Dead Wrong	59
Day 60	There Is a Way That Seems Right	60
Day 61	Power of Words	61

Day 62	Love to Eat?	62
Day 63	Move It or Lose It	63
Day 64	Trust God's Design	64
Day 65	Hopeless?	65
Day 66	Too Much of a Good Thing	66
Day 67	Can You See?	67
Day 68	Are You Chasing the Wind?	68
Day 69	As a Twig Is Bent, So Grows the Tree	69
Day 70	Love Letter	70
Day 71	Have We Made Modern Medicine an Idol?	71
Day 72	Power of Prayer	72
Day 73	Jesus Loves You at the Cellular Level!	73
Day 74	He Is a Generational God	74
Day 75	We Need Jesus	75
Day 76	Mother's Milk	76
Day 77	You Are Not Alone	77
Day 78	Before You Were Even Born	78
Day 79	Choose the Things of God	79
Day 80	Do Not Fear	80
Day 81	A New Heart, Stomach, and Liver	81
Day 82	Dry Bones	82
Day 83	The Daniel Fast	83
Day 84	Facing the Fiery Furnace	84
Day 85	Not So Fast	85
Day 86	Wait on Your God	86
Day 87	Come Back to God	87
Day 88	Dream Dreams	88
Day 89	Giver of Life	89
Day 90	Urgency	90
Day 91	You Can Run, but You Can't Hide	91
Day 92	Tell Me What I Want to Hear	92
Day 93	A God Like You	93
Day 94	The Lord Is Good, Just, and Fair	94

Day 95	How Long, Lord, Must I Call for Help?............ 95
Day 96	He Is Mighty to Save 96
Day 97	God First..................................... 97
Day 98	The Future.................................... 98
Day 99	Are You Robbing God? 99
Day 100	The Faithful Few—the Remnant 100
Day 101	With Child From the Holy Spirit 101
Day 102	Baptism by Fire 102
Day 103	Temptation 103
Day 104	Jesus Heals the Sick 104
Day 105	Let Your Light Shine! 105
Day 106	Anger 106
Day 107	Fasting 107
Day 108	Treasures in Heaven 108
Day 109	Open the Eyes............................... 109
Day 110	Do Not Be Anxious........................... 110
Day 111	The Incurable Disease of Leprosy—Gone 111
Day 112	You Are a Cancer Killer! 112
Day 113	Healed by the Faith of Someone Else 113
Day 114	Jesus Heals Even In-laws 114
Day 115	Jesus Calms the Storm 115
Day 116	Not Everyone Will Be Happy About Your Healing 116
Day 117	Rise 117
Day 118	It Is Never Too Late.......................... 118
Day 119	I Was Blind, but Now I See.................... 119
Day 120	Dealing With Demons 120
Day 121	He Had Compassion on Them 121
Day 122	He Knows the Hairs on Your Head! 122
Day 123	Healing on the Sabbath....................... 123
Day 124	He Gave Thanks and Then Fed All Five Thousand!............................... 124
Day 125	Water Walker 125

Day 126   Just a Touch 126

Day 127   Do You Have a Heart Condition? 127

Day 128   Persistence Pays. 128

Day 129   God Is Enough 129

Day 130   Another Supernatural Buffet 130

Day 131   Things of God or Things of Man. 131

Day 132   Move Mountains. 132

Day 133   Protect Our Children! 133

Day 134   With God *All* Things Are Possible. 134

Day 135   Two Blind Men—Another Miracle. 135

Day 136   Full-Faith Prayers. 136

Day 137   God's Design Beats Man's Every Time. 137

Day 138   Get to the Cause. 138

Day 139   But Some Doubted 139

Day 140   More Harm Than Good? 140

Day 141   Even Jesus Enjoyed Exercise—
He Walked on Water! 141

Day 142   Be Honest With Jesus—
He Knows Already Anyway! 142

Day 143   The Healing Power of Spit 143

Day 144   The Butterfly. 144

Day 145   Love. 145

Day 146   Wake Up—The Truth Is Right in Front of You! 146

Day 147   Leap for Joy. 147

Day 148   How Many Germs Do You Think Were
in the Manger? 148

Day 149   Rejected 149

Day 150   Break the Nets! 150

Day 151   Sometimes You Have to Cut a Hole
in the Roof!. 151

Day 152   New (Wine)skins 152

Day 153   You Can Tell a Tree by Its Fruit 153

Day 154   It Is Never Too Late. 154

Day 155 Can You Wait Just a Second, Jesus?.............. 155
Day 156 Don't Miss Him 156
Day 157 The Power of Prayer 157
Day 158 The Eye Gate................................ 158
Day 159 Frankenfood................................ 159
Day 160 You Are More Valuable Than the Sparrows 160
Day 161 Do You Really Need That Soda? 161
Day 162 Much Is Asked............................... 162
Day 163 Jesus Saw Her............................... 163
Day 164 Jesus Heals................................. 164
Day 165 Count the Costs 165
Day 166 Cleanse the Temple........................... 166
Day 167 Jesus Heals an Ear!........................... 167
Day 168 The Veil Was Torn............................ 168
Day 169 Water Into Wine 169
Day 170 "Do You Want to Get Well?" 170
Day 171 He Is the Bread of Life 171
Day 172 The Truth Hurts.............................. 172
Day 173 My Glory Is Nothing 173
Day 174 For the Glory of God 174
Day 175 God Is the Creator of Life!..................... 175
Day 176 Whom Are You Listening To?.................... 176
Day 177 Lazarus, Come Out............................ 177
Day 178 Peace of My Heart 178
Day 179 The Vine 179
Day 180 Don't Bury Your Head in the Sand 180
Day 181 Doubting Thomas 181
Day 182 Feed My Sheep.............................. 182
Day 183 The Holy Spirit Comes 183
Day 184 Healing in the Name of Jesus 184
Day 185 Obey God, Not Man.......................... 185
Day 186 The Apostles Healed Many..................... 186
Day 187 Do You Believe in Miracles? 187

Day 188	Sit Up Straight!	188
Day 189	Stoned to Death	189
Day 190	There Was Great Joy in the City	190
Day 191	Saul Is Changed	191
Day 192	Roll Up Your Mat.	192
Day 193	Another Resurrection.	193
Day 194	You've Got This!.	194
Day 195	Even in Prison.	195
Day 196	Move!	196
Day 197	Just a Touch	197
Day 198	A Tragic Accident Redeemed	198
Day 199	Snakebites and More Healings.	199
Day 200	Peace and Joy	200
Day 201	More Sinning = More Grace?	201
Day 202	Live by the Spirit	202
Day 203	The Holy Spirit Intercedes	203
Day 204	But That's Not Fair.	204
Day 205	Mic Drop!.	205
Day 206	Renew Your Mind	206
Day 207	Many Parts, One Body.	207
Day 208	Some Practical Teaching	208
Day 209	Trigger Warning for Germaphobes	209
Day 210	Man's Wisdom?.	210
Day 211	Keep It Simple	211
Day 212	Eyes to See	212
Day 213	Wisdom From the Spirit	213
Day 214	Feed Your Brain!	214
Day 215	The Temple of the Holy Spirit, Part 1	215
Day 216	The Temple of the Holy Spirit, Part 2	216
Day 217	The Temple of the Holy Spirit, Part 3	217
Day 218	Is Food an Idol to You?	218
Day 219	Flee Evil	219
Day 220	Give God the Glory	220

Day 221	Food as a Stronghold?........................ 221
Day 222	Gifts of the Spirit............................. 222
Day 223	All Together Now 223
Day 224	Body of Christ 224
Day 225	Love Is..................................... 225
Day 226	Be a Liver 226
Day 227	The God of All Comfort 227
Day 228	Blinded by the Light 228
Day 229	Living by Faith, Not by Sight 229
Day 230	A New Creation 230
Day 231	And You Think You Have Had It Rough 231
Day 232	Be Careful Whom You Yoke With............... 232
Day 233	Purify...................................... 233
Day 234	Godly Sorrow 234
Day 235	Do You Have a Generous Heart?............... 235
Day 236	Reap What You Sow 236
Day 237	Take Every Thought Captive 237
Day 238	His Grace Is Sufficient 238
Day 239	Are You Seeking Approval of Man or God?...... 239
Day 240	Fourteen Years.............................. 240
Day 241	"I No Longer Live" 241
Day 242	Who Bewitched You?......................... 242
Day 243	Known by God 243
Day 244	Freedom.................................... 244
Day 245	Is Your Fishbowl Dirty?....................... 245
Day 246	Wise Words................................. 246
Day 247	Life by the Spirit............................. 247
Day 248	Today Is the Day! 248
Day 249	Do Not Grow Weary in Doing Good Work....... 249
Day 250	The Gospel: Remember *Who* and *Whose* You Are...250
Day 251	For the Praise of His Glory.................... 251
Day 252	Even When We Were Dead in Our Transgressions 252

Day 253   Saved by Grace—God's Gift 253
Day 254   God Prepared Beforehand 254
Day 255   Blood 255
Day 256   A Powerful Prayer 256
Day 257   Worthy of the Call! 257
Day 258   A Measure of Grace............................258
Day 259   Grow Up 259
Day 260   New Life......................................260
Day 261   Renew Your Mind 261
Day 262   Forgiveness 262
Day 263   Be Imitators of Christ........................263
Day 264   Be Wise 264
Day 265   The Full Armor of God 265
Day 266   Pray in the Spirit 266
Day 267   Carry It to Completion 267
Day 268   Even in Chains................................268
Day 269   To Live Is Christ, to Die Is Gain 269
Day 270   Do Nothing Out of Selfish Ambition............270
Day 271   Shine Like Stars 271
Day 272   The Surpassing Greatness of Knowing Christ 272
Day 273   Straining Toward What Is Ahead 273
Day 274   Especially When It Is Difficult 274
Day 275   Peace That Surpasses Understanding. 275
Day 276   Pray..276
Day 277   As a Man Thinks... 277
Day 278   I Can Do All Things Through Christ
          Who Gives Me Strength 278
Day 279   Live a Worthy Life............................279
Day 280   Jesus Holds Us All Together...................280
Day 281   Christ in You, the Hope of Glory.............. 281
Day 282   Need Some Good Advice?........................282
Day 283   Don't Be Fooled...............................283
Day 284   Eyes Up 284

Day 285	What Needs to Die?............................285
Day 286	Peace of Christ................................286
Day 287	Work for the Lord 287
Day 288	Seasoned With Salt 288
Day 289	Faith, Hope, and Love 289
Day 290	Do Not Put Out the Spirit's Fire.................290
Day 291	Test Everything................................291
Day 292	They Refused to Love Truth.....................292
Day 293	Get Busy.....................................293
Day 294	Christ Jesus Came to Save Sinners 294
Day 295	Manage Your Family 295
Day 296	Some Will Abandon the Faith...................296
Day 297	Godliness With Contentment...................297
Day 298	Fight the Good Fight of Faith....................298
Day 299	A Warning to the Rich 299
Day 300	A Spirit of Power..............................300
Day 301	Flee Evil Desires of Youth.......................301
Day 302	People Will Be Lovers of Themselves—
	Selfie Culture.................................302
Day 303	All Scripture Is God Breathed 303
Day 304	But I Like It!...................................304
Day 305	Poured Out...................................305
Day 306	At One Time, We Too Were Foolish..............306
Day 307	Regeneration.................................307
Day 308	Refreshed the Hearts..........................308
Day 309	Testified by Signs, Wonders, and Miracles 309
Day 310	Are You Afraid of Death?.......................310
Day 311	Rest 311
Day 312	The Word of God Is Alive 312
Day 313	Approach the Throne of Grace With
	Confidence...................................313
Day 314	Are You Mature?..............................314
Day 315	Faith 315

Day 316   Faith, Continued 316
Day 317   The Weight of Sin 317
Day 318   Run the Race 318
Day 319   The Author of Our Faith 319
Day 320   The Discipline of God......................... 320
Day 321   Refrain 321
Day 322   A Consuming Fire 322
Day 323   Entertaining Angels........................... 323
Day 324   Count It Pure Joy 324
Day 325   Be Wise!..................................... 325
Day 326   God Will Never Tempt You 326
Day 327   Are You Deceiving Yourself? 327
Day 328   Even the Demons Believe That................. 328
Day 329   Can a Fig Tree Bear Olives? 329
Day 330   Wisdom? 330
Day 331   Submit Yourselves to God 331
Day 332   Your Life Is a Mist 332
Day 333   Sin of Omission 333
Day 334   A Warning Against Self-Indulging 334
Day 335   Just a Little Patience 335
Day 336   Anoint Them With Oil......................... 336
Day 337   Refined by Fire............................... 337
Day 338   Be Holy Because I Am Holy 338
Day 339   Taste and See That the Lord Is Good............ 339
Day 340   Abstain From the Passions of the Flesh........... 340
Day 341   Zealous for God 341
Day 342   Your Body Is a Gift 342
Day 343   Cast All Your Anxiety on Him 343
Day 344   Slow Down................................... 344
Day 345   Everything You Need 345
Day 346   Beware of Counterfeits........................ 346
Day 347   A Man Is a Slave to Whatever Has
            Mastered Him 347

Day 348	Nothing but the Blood of Jesus	348
Day 349	The Man Who Does the Will of God Lives Forever	349
Day 350	Children of God Should Not Be This Sick!	350
Day 351	God Loves His Children	351
Day 352	What Do You Confess?	352
Day 353	Greater Is He That Is in You	353
Day 354	Love	354
Day 355	His Commands Are Not Burdensome	355
Day 356	Believe	356
Day 357	Face to Face	357
Day 358	Walking in Truth	358
Day 359	Contend for the Faith	359
Day 360	The Time Is Now	360
Day 361	Holy	361
Day 362	Hindsight Is Twenty-Twenty	362
Day 363	Drugs Don't Heal—Jesus Does	363
Day 364	The Rider on the White Horse	364
Day 365	Water of Life	365
	Appendix: Nervous System	366
	Notes	367
	About the Author	378

PREFACE

Years ago I read *God and Money* by John Cortines and Gregory Baumer, and I thought, "Someone should write a book about God and health." I often thought about doing so, but I felt unqualified. Even though I have had many experiences with the healing power of Jesus both personally and professionally as a chiropractor for twenty years, I still hoped someone else would write it.

Years went by. Then I was awakened at 4 a.m. in midsummer 2022, and the Lord told me, "Write a 365-day devotional from Genesis to Revelation through the lens of My healing power." For three months I would write from 5 a.m. to 7 a.m. I wrote everything by hand and filled two journals with daily devotionals. I assumed I would simply self-publish the book and encourage my patients and those looking to understand God's healing power and wellness to read it. A friend introduced me to Charisma Media, but I assumed I had no chance of being picked up as an author. Yet God had other plans. They thought the book would be a blessing, and we moved forward.

My prayer for you is that as you make your way through these pages, one day at a time, asking yourself some tough questions and being challenged on your views of health and healing, something supernatural will happen—that fear will be broken, diseases healed, and generations of addiction and mental health challenges crushed. I pray the power of Jesus through these selected scriptures sets you free.

I believe God told me to write this book, and I was obedient. Now the ball is in your court. I pray that as you read these words, ponder the questions, and put new practices into action, you will discover that your body was designed to heal.

INTRODUCTION

JESUS SAVED ME at thirteen years old. The next Sunday, as we were walking into church, my mom said, "Tell Joni (a family friend) what happened last week." So I got puffed up and told her I was saved, expecting her to say something congratulatory. Instead, Joni stopped, looked at me, and said, "Well, you did the easy part."

Those words have rung in my head for over thirty years. I have experienced the healing power of Jesus in my own personal health, and as a practicing chiropractor for twenty years with more than fifteen thousand patient cases, I have seen a lot. One of the things I have seen is an unfortunate increase in the idol worship of man-made health care. America has become the most "medicalized" nation in the world. Yet we are getting sicker. We lead the world in prescription drug use and health-care spending and rank high in obesity rates and cancer-related deaths. I have noticed the church at large rarely discusses health and wellness care; it is almost taboo in many churches. God created us in His likeness and image, yet we don't seem to take much responsibility for caring for our bodies appropriately.

I pray this book changes that for you. I pray it helps you ask questions you may never have asked yourself before. I pray it helps you think critically and consider what the Scriptures do and don't say regarding health and healing.

This book will likely challenge some of the assumptions you have about health and healing. Take it one day at a time. That is how God designed us to care for our health as well— one day at a time, 365 days a year. He designed you to heal.

Day 1
IN THE BEGINNING, GOD

In the beginning God created the heavens and the earth.
—GENESIS 1:1

GOD MADE EVERYTHING out of nothing. We humans have never made a single cell, yet scientists estimate that we have anywhere from 37 to 100 trillion of them! There is an old joke about a scientist who challenged God to a human-making competition. He said he had figured it out and could do a better job than God. But when the scientist scooped up some dirt to begin his project, God said, "Make your own dirt; I did!"

This exposes the pride and arrogance we often have toward God and His creation. We are called to steward and care for His creation, not try to be superior to Him as the creator. His design is perfect.

TAKE HEART

Nothing is too hard for the God who made everything. Do you have more faith in mankind or in God? Imagine what it would have been like to be there in the beginning when God created everything. My encouragement for you is to remember you are made by God.

TAKE ACTION

Take a few minutes to think about or look up some beautiful natural wonders, such as the Grand Canyon, Victoria Falls, or the Blue Ridge Mountains. Let them remind of you of the awesome creativity of the God who made you.

Day 2
DIVINE DESIGN

*Then God said, "Let us make mankind in our image, in our
likeness, so that they may rule over the fish in the sea and
the birds in the sky, over the livestock and all the wild animals, and over all the creatures that move along the ground."
So God created mankind in his own image, in the image of
God he created them; male and female he created them.*
—GENESIS 1:26–27

GOD DESIGNED US in His image. This truth is a game
changer. It can eliminate any fear, doubt, or worry when
you realize and believe how much God loves you and just how
incredibly and divinely you are created.

TAKE HEART

You *matter*. You were divinely created by the greatest Creator,
Doctor, Designer in all of history. You are a masterpiece, created in the likeness and image of the Master. Meditate on that
for a moment. Soak on that. Preach it to yourself every day. It
is a critical daily reminder.

TAKE ACTION

Is this enough to challenge any doubts about your value to
God? To be encouraged in your divine design? You are literally made in the image of God. Go look in a mirror today at
all the parts of your body. What do you think? The way you
were designed is so incredible!

Day 3
HE IS A GOD OF MORE THAN ENOUGH!

God blessed them and said to them, "Be fruitful and mul-
tiply, and replenish the earth and subdue it. Rule over
the fish of the sea and over the birds of the air and
over every living thing that moves on the earth."
—GENESIS 1:28, MEV

HERE IS AN amazing fact: A man can produce several million new sperm each day—and enough within about two
months to repopulate the earth![1] We know that ultimately
God is the creator of life, but it is amazing the potential He
puts in us. It is so like God to overprovide for us in ways that
are almost unbelievable.

The saddest places on earth are cemeteries—not because of
the dead bodies but because of the lost potential. Don't waste
what God has given you.

TAKE HEART

Are you living up to the potential God invested in you?

TAKE ACTION

Choose one thing to do that will help you reach the potential
God gave you.

Day 4
SABBATH

*By the seventh day God had finished the work he had been
doing; so on the seventh day he rested from all his work.*
—GENESIS 2:2

GOD DESIGNED REST. He didn't need to rest (He's God!),
but He knows what is perfect and needed for us. Rest is
as important as work. Think about sleep. It is the great equal-
izer: every person sleeps, from the president to a newborn
baby. Why did God create us to need sleep? Rest? Divine rest?

Did you know that a significant amount of healing happens
during sleep? Memories get imprinted, cells repair, growth
happens—all while you are asleep.

TAKE HEART

Do you honor the Sabbath? Do you practice Sabbath? Why or
why not? It was good enough for God, and you are created in
His image. Since He chose to rest, you need to do that too! He
created the Sabbath, a time He gave us to rest in Him.

TAKE ACTION

Take one day and rest. Add one hour to your sleep.

Day 5
HE IS THE BREATH IN OUR LUNGS

*Then the LORD God formed a man from the dust of
the ground and breathed into his nostrils the breath
of life, and the man became a living being.*
—GENESIS 2:7

GOD'S DESIGN IS incredible. Some researchers say that together, your lungs have the surface area about the size of a tennis court.[1] *Mind blown!* If you struggle with trusting the body God created for you—or trusting God—it often helps to study and learn amazing facts about the body or aspects of God to help increase your faith. One of my goals for this book is to increase your faith in God by showing you through the body He gave you how amazing and trustworthy He is.

TAKE HEART

God has shown himself to be worthy of our trust. Remember, He created you. He knows the number of hairs on your head— no other doctor knows that. God is the great physician.

TAKE ACTION

Take a few minutes to just examine your body, your hands, your fingers—how they move, grip, and turn. The divine design of your body is breathtaking!

Day 6
WORK IT...WITH OTHERS

*The LORD God took the man and put him in the
Garden of Eden to work it and take care of it....The
LORD God said, "It is not good for the man to be
alone. I will make a helper suitable for him."*
—GENESIS 2:15, 18

WE ARE CREATED and divinely called to do work. And
we are designed for relationship—first with God, and
second with others.

Many studies on longevity have shown the importance
of purpose (work)[1] and relationships.[2] Many people without
these things die soon after their retirement. We often resent or
complain about work, yet we are created *by God* to do work!

TAKE HEART

Do you look at your work as a divine calling? Do you recognize that you were created to do work? Are you lonely? Do
you have friends—not social media "friends" but real people
you can talk, pray, laugh, and cry with? It matters more than
you think!

TAKE ACTION

Schedule a lunch with a friend, a family member, or your
spouse.

Day 7
WHAT DID HE SAY? DID HE REALLY SAY THAT?

Now the serpent was more crafty than any of the wild animals the LORD God had made. He said to the woman, "Did God really say, 'You must not eat from any tree in the garden'?"
—GENESIS 3:1

OH HOW QUICKLY we forget and question God's truths, promises, and ways. We want the hack, the shortcut, and often we want "to be like God." The amazing thing is, He allows us to choose. Every day we make choices that are good or evil, healthy or unhealthy:

- We decide whether we are going to pray.
- We decide what to eat.
- We choose the words we speak.
- We decide to log on to social media.

What direction are each of these choices and decisions leading us in? Are they drawing us closer to God or farther away?

TAKE HEART

Which is better: your way (the flesh) or God's way?

TAKE ACTION

Just say no. Most of the changes we need to make are not things to do; they are things to *stop* doing. What do you need to say no to or remove from your life?

Day 8
120

Then the LORD said, "My Spirit will not con-
tend with humans forever, for they are mortal; their
days will be a hundred and twenty years."
—GENESIS 6:3

THE LORD'S DESIGN (which science has validated) is that cells have about 120 years of life to them.[1] Then why do so many of us fall short by forty to fifty years?

When we go against God's natural design for life, there are consequences. Cause and effect—we reap what we sow.

When it comes down to it, a live body and a dead body generally have the same parts. Each has a brain, heart, lungs, liver, and so on—but one is alive and the other is dead. It's about life versus death.

TAKE HEART

God is the creator and giver of life. You are designed for 120 years. Are you doing your part? Are you living a life and life-style aligned with God's plans and design?

TAKE ACTION

Challenge some of your views and assumptions about life, health, and longevity. What do you think about living to 120? Are you "running your race" well? Whom have you allowed to set your expectations about life and health: culture or God?

Day 9
THE RAINBOW

*I have set my rainbow in the clouds, and it will be the
sign of the covenant between me and the earth.*
—GENESIS 9:13

How cool is it to think about God making the first
rainbow? Can you imagine hearing God describe it?
And then, *boom!* The most astonishing rainbow in the sky
formed. Amazing.

God is a God who keeps His word. He's worth trusting.
He's perfect. And His ways are perfect.

Do you trust Him? Do you see His rainbow and remember
His love and promises? Oh how quickly we forget and complain. His promises are as true today as ever. Sometimes
we need to be reminded. We need to see the rainbow. The
promise. The truth.

TAKE HEART

God is trustworthy in all ways—spiritually, physically, emotionally, financially, and relationally.

TAKE ACTION

Keep your eyes and heart open for rainbows, for the truths
God has spoken. Take a picture of the next rainbow you see.
God made it for you, and it carries His promises!

Day 10
ARE YOU WILLING?

Then God said, "Take your son, your only son, whom you love—Isaac—and go to the region of Moriah. Sacrifice him there as a burnt offering on a mountain I will show you."
—GENESIS 22:2

THIS IS ONE of the most intense stories from the Old Testament. Any parent who has read it can imagine the tension and emotion. Thank God there is a happy ending! The Lord provided a substitute at the last second—but not until Abraham showed he was willing to do whatever the Lord asked him to do.

When it comes to our lives, health, and lifestyle choices, what do we need to sacrifice? One of my patients loved Coke and couldn't quit drinking it. Then I encouraged her to quit for God. That perspective opened her mind and heart to think about Coke in a whole new way. As an expression of worship and obedience to God, she stopped drinking it.

TAKE HEART

Sacrifice is important! Giving up junk food, alcohol, tobacco, or the like is certainly not as difficult as sacrificing one of your children, but it can still be challenging. What is God asking you to give up?

TAKE ACTION

Skip breakfast just once. Do it for God.

Day 11
GRUMBLING IN THE DESERT

*The Israelites said to them, "If only we had died by the
LORD's hand in Egypt! There we sat around pots of meat
and ate all the food we wanted, but you have brought us
out into this desert to starve this entire assembly to death."*
—EXODUS 16:3

IMAGINE THAT YOU have been freed from terrible slavery and have just seen one of the greatest miracles—the parting of the Red Sea. Yet a few days later you are asking to be a slave again!

Old habits die hard. Make no mistake, changing your lifestyle and habits can be difficult. You will need the Holy Spirit's help to do it. There will be days when you just want to return to the slavery of your old life. But God has promised that He is with you. He will provide a way.

Lean on Him. Pray to Him. Be honest. Show your struggle—He already knows anyway.

TAKE HEART

Freedom is not free! Take responsibility for your actions and choices. Don't blame anyone. Don't blame your genetics. And don't blame God.

TAKE ACTION

Are you grumbling? Find ways to turn your pain to praise, and expect God to deliver manna from heaven. He is Jehovah Jireh—our provider!

Day 12

SOMETIMES WE NEED TO FOLLOW THE RECIPE

As for the perfume which you will make, you
may not make it for yourselves using the same
recipe. It must be holy for the LORD to you.
—EXODUS 30:37, MEV

JUICE (IN THIS order) ten celery stalks, one to two cucumbers, two bunches kale, two bunches spinach, one Granny Smith apple (optional), half a broccoli stalk, one lemon (peeled), a quarter-inch ring fresh ginger root (peeled), and seven to ten stalks of parsley (add this last because it tends to bind in the juicer). This is the exact green juice recipe we used to care for my dad after he was diagnosed with stage IV cancer and given two weeks to live. He lived on only this for ten days straight. It was very powerful for his healing. He was able to reverse his cancer using holistic methods. I watched my dad's health transform before my eyes.

You don't have to wait until you have a terminal illness to change your lifestyle. Use this recipe as a boost to your health!

TAKE HEART

Is your lifestyle building health or leading to disease? Are you nourishing your mind, body, and spirit or burdening them?

TAKE ACTION

Try a juice fast for one to three days. You can use this recipe or find premade juices. Just be careful to avoid juices with lots of sugar.

Day 13
AMERICAN IDOL

Then the LORD said to Moses, "Go down, because your people, whom you brought up out of Egypt, have become corrupt. They have been quick to turn away from what I commanded them and have made themselves an idol cast in the shape of a calf."
—EXODUS 32:7–8

OH HOW SOME things never change. The human condition is something! We think we will never fall for the trap again. However, even as good, God-fearing people, when we don't get what we want when we want it, we pervert the Lord's word and sprinkle in some things we miss and want. We begin to worship new idols—often culturally acceptable ones—so we don't look silly.

We may stop drinking soda but start indulging in a new "guilty pleasure." We like to find shiny new things that make us feel good—but we don't like to call them idols. We allow these idols to sneak back into our lives. Yet the Lord clearly shows how He feels about idols.

TAKE HEART

Have you created new idols? Have you gotten off Facebook but logged on to Instagram? Have you said no to five Diet Cokes a day but now drink five Starbucks beverages a day instead?

TAKE ACTION

Review and audit. Get honest about where you have let selfishness and comfort sneak back into your life. What can you not imagine losing? Maybe that's an idol.

Day 14
ARE YOU RADIATING?

*So when Aaron and all the children of Israel
saw Moses, amazingly, the skin of his face shone,
and they were afraid to come near him.*
—EXODUS 34:30, MEV

YOUR SKIN IS the largest organ of your body, and it is a full-blown miracle. Something as simple as your skin sweats, heals itself, grows hair, detoxes you, protects you from outside elements, and constantly regenerates. *Amazing!*

TAKE HEART

When is the last time you thought about how amazing your skin is? Or do you just take it for granted? How many other things do you think God does to sustain us that we never think about?

TAKE ACTION

Look at your hand, your arm, or your fingertip. Get close to your mirror, and look at your face. Your skin is a wonder. And remember, in all of history there have never been two fingerprints that are the same! The God who designed all this even knows the number of hairs on your head.

Day 15

DO NOT...

You shall keep My statutes.
—LEVITICUS 19:19, MEV

MUCH OF THE Book of Leviticus could introduce today's theme, because it is where God established His laws about morality and purity that were to set the Israelites apart from other nations. We don't like to be told what we cannot do, especially in today's culture of self, "good vibes only," and "follow your heart." Nor do we like to be told what is right and wrong. When many of us were children, our parents warned us about doing harmful things. Sometimes we did them anyway and learned the hard way.

Rules are not meant to confuse or hurt us; they are meant to protect. Some of us have the wrong perspective on God's laws, not realizing they are for our benefit. How blessed we are to have God's laws recorded for us! We can celebrate.

TAKE HEART

Are you resisting what is right? Why? Talk to God about it.

TAKE ACTION

What is one habit you already know that you need to stop? Go one day without it as a form of worship to God.

Day 16

WHERE DID EVERYBODY GO?

*The ground under them split apart and the earth opened its
mouth and swallowed them and their households, and all those
associated with Korah, together with their possessions. They
went down alive into the realm of the dead, with everything they
owned; the earth closed over them, and they perished and were
gone from the community. At their cries, all the Israelites around
them fled, shouting, "The earth is going to swallow us too!"*
—NUMBERS 16:31–34

WHEN YOU BEGIN to live a life that is set apart, some
people will not celebrate and congratulate you. They
may get jealous, angry, and resentful—and these are just
people you considered "friends"!

As you begin to change habits that have become idols or
remove things that have not edified your life (such as social
media, television, sinful life choices, etc.), some people may
not like the new you. This is when staying focused on God
and His ways becomes essential.

TAKE HEART

Are you focusing on pleasing God or others? Stay the course.
Your new ways will bring new people into your life. Have you
been afraid of what others will think? Are you afraid of what
God thinks?

TAKE ACTION

Say no to the people you need to and yes to some new ones.
When is the last time you went to church? Maybe it is time.

Day 17
BLESSED FOR OBEDIENCE

All these blessings will come on you and accompany you if you obey the LORD your God.
—DEUTERONOMY 28:2

FOLLOWING THE WAYS of God is not restrictive and punitive. It means *freedom* and *blessing*. All He wants is what is best for us, and He made incredible promises to us about the blessing of living in alignment with His ways.

Reframe God's ways. If you wanted to be a great athlete and found out the greatest coach ever was going to mentor you, how would you feel? I assure you that you would be excited—and maybe even a little intimidated. But what an opportunity! Sure, following the coach's instructions would be hard some days, but it would also bring lots of blessings. This is similar to the Holy Spirit in our lives. Following His lead may be difficult at times, but what an amazing gift and opportunity!

TAKE HEART

Are you willing to let God be your leader, coach, counselor, advocate, healer, and provider?

TAKE ACTION

Think of one or two areas in your life where you have not sought God's wisdom (money, relationships, health, etc.). Today is a great day to talk to God about those areas.

Day 18
DIGEST THE WORD OF GOD

*Of Benjamin he said: The beloved of the LORD will
dwell in safety by Him, and the LORD will protect him
all day long; he will dwell between His shoulders.*
—DEUTERONOMY 33:12, MEV

HERE IS AN amazing fact about the body God made for you: Stomach acid is strong enough to dissolve metal, but your body continually secretes a substance to stop your stomach from digesting itself. Incredible! If your body stopped doing this simple yet amazing thing for a length of time, you would die. *Thank You, Jesus, for being my protector.*

TAKE HEART

How many other astonishing facts about our bodies do you think we have yet to even discover? Does this amaze you? Humble you? Encourage you?

TAKE ACTION

Today, when you are eating, consider the countless things happening to allow that meal to be digested. Give thanks!

Day 19
HE WILL NEVER LEAVE
OR FORSAKE YOU

*No one will be able to stand against you all the
days of your life. As I was with Moses, so I will be
with you; I will never leave you nor forsake you.*
—Joshua 1:5

THE GREATEST THING about God's promises is that they
are *true*, no matter what—even when they don't seem true.
This is really important to remember. If we don't trust or have
faith, not only will we quit or give up, but we may blame God
or lose faith. This can often lead to getting sucked into the
latest fads of the day: the newest diet, drug, vaccine, therapy,
test, etc.

Why are we so apt to give up on God and run to human
wisdom? The sad irony of this tendency is incredible and
telling. The One who made us and knows us better than we
know ourselves died for us and said He would never leave or
forsake us. Yet we can be so fickle with Him. We want a genie
in a bottle, but Jesus is not a genie. He is God.

TAKE HEART

Align your perspective with the truth. Have you come under
the authority of a mighty God? Why not?

TAKE ACTION

Review your day. Where is your faith: in God or in mankind?

Day 20
AND THE WALLS CAME DOWN!

When the trumpets sounded, the army shouted, and at the sound of the trumpet, when the men gave a loud shout, the wall collapsed; so everyone charged straight in, and they took the city.
—JOSHUA 6:20

MANY TIMES, WE may be doing the right thing but not seeing the results we want yet. It's like we're on day 6 and the walls of Jericho are still standing.

As we change our lifestyles, we often want immediate results. When we don't get what we're looking for right away, we can come to the wrong conclusions. But what if Joshua and the Israelites had stopped marching on day 6? The walls of Jericho fell on day 7.

TAKE HEART

What areas of change in your life or faith have you stopped too soon? Keep moving and blowing the horn! God will bless it. You may not always see the results as fast as you want. Sometimes you may feel like you are walking in circles, but what you are really doing is shaking the foundations. Breakthrough is coming!

TAKE ACTION

Commit to making one change for thirty straight days. It could be something like drinking a glass of water every morning, taking a fifteen-minute walk each day, or making time for daily prayer.

DESIGNED TO HEAL

Day 21
PRAYERS THAT STOP TIME

*There has never been a day like it before or since, a
day when the LORD listened to a human being.*
—JOSHUA 10:14

WHEN JOSHUA PRAYED for the sun to stand still and it
did, the world was never the same. Do you pray "sun
stand still" prayers in situations that seem impossible? Have
you prayed about your health and others' health? What about
habits? Or mental health?

Do you want to lose weight? Have you prayed?

Do you need to start exercising? Have you prayed?

Are you depressed or anxious? Have you prayed?

Do you have a diagnosed disease? Have you prayed?

Also, Scripture tells us to pray for one another. Have you
asked others to pray for you? Have you prayed for them? Have
you had people lay hands on you? Have you been anointed
with oil by church elders?

TAKE HEART

Think about an area of your health or lifestyle you are struggling with. Have you prayed about it? How often? Do you still
believe that God can heal you and set you free?

TAKE ACTION

Pray for your and others' healing. Pray bold and audacious
prayers. Do it *now*!

Day 22

DON'T TELL ME WHAT TO DO

In those days Israel had no king; everyone did as they saw fit.
—JUDGES 17:6

MANY, IF NOT all, of us have resisted authority at some level. We don't want to be told what to do. This is human nature, from as far back as the Garden—and it reveals why we desperately need God. Left to our own human devices (indulging self and the flesh), we tend to destroy ourselves. It may feel good for a while. It may even feel like "freedom." But we become slaves to sin and the flesh.

In today's world, as in every era of history, we need to surrender to God. We need to surrender everything: our lives, our health, our kids, our work, our marriages, etc.

TAKE HEART

Do you listen to God, or are you just doing as you see fit? How is it going?

TAKE ACTION

What is one area you need to give to God? Money? Marriage? A habitual sin? Begin to surrender it now.

Day 23

BE AN INFLUENCER

*The women living there said, "Naomi has a
son!" And they named him Obed. He was the
father of Jesse, the father of David.*
—RUTH 4:17

Ruth's obedience and generous heart toward her mother-in-law (yes, mother-in-law) led to a cascade of effects that put her in the lineage of the Messiah, even though she would not live to see Jesus in person. Sure, living in obedience and stewarding what God has provided for us benefit us personally, but often, if not always, there is more to the story—much of which we may never see.

Pioneering chiropractor B. J. Palmer is quoted as saying, "We never know how far reaching something we may think, say or do today will affect the lives of millions tomorrow." Your choices have distant reverberations—even for your children's children's children. In other words, your life and choices produce ripple effects like those of a stone thrown into a lake. Are you leaving good ripples?

TAKE HEART

Are you creating a divine legacy?

TAKE ACTION

Spend some time dreaming of the future generations and reflecting on where you come from. Can you see good patterns? Bad patterns? What strongholds do you need to break?

WHAT GOES ON GOES IN

*Then Samuel took a flask of olive oil and poured it
on Saul's head and kissed him, saying, "Has not the
LORD anointed you ruler over his inheritance?*
—1 SAMUEL 10:1

THERE ARE BOTH good things and toxic things to put on our bodies. Most people don't think much about the chemicals they use on their skin or the toxic health effects these products can cause. Yet the chemicals we put on our skin penetrate into our bodies quickly and can have massive effects on our health—everything from allergic reactions to cancer. Most chemicals used in makeup, sunscreen, hand sanitizer, cleaning products, and personal hygiene items have not been properly tested for their short- or long-term effects. While you are trying to enhance your beauty and smell good, you may be making yourself sick. Oftentimes less is more. Most of the cleaning around our house is done with vinegar and baking soda. Look at the products you are using and see if you can remove any, or at least reduce some.

TAKE HEART

Consider how many different chemicals you use on a daily basis—in personal care products, in air fresheners, at work, and so on. Are you surprised by the sheer number?

TAKE ACTION

Go to EWG.org, and look up some of your products. Notice what toxins are in them and what effects they can have.

Day 25
WHAT IS YOUR ANOINTING?

Then the LORD said, "Rise and anoint him; this is the one."
—1 SAMUEL 16:12

DAVID WAS NOT the cream of the crop in the world's eyes. He was just the little, forgotten shepherd boy, but he was the one destined and anointed to be king. (It took about fifteen to twenty years before he actually assumed the throne, but the anointing was on him the whole time.)

Now you may not have had a prophet come to your home, pull you from a field, and pour oil on your head. But know this: God created you specifically, for a specific time, with specific plans and purposes. That is an anointing from the God who made you.

TAKE HEART

Do you feel anointed? Is it hard for you to believe God has anointed *you*? Have you prayed about what God has anointed you to do?

TAKE ACTION

God has plans for your divine purpose. Pray right now and ask Him to reveal it to you. Walk in your anointing. The implications are for now and all eternity.

Day 26
WHAT'S YOUR GOLIATH?

David said to the Philistine, "You come against me
with sword and spear and javelin, but I come against
you in the name of the LORD Almighty, the God of
the armies of Israel, whom you have defied.
—1 SAMUEL 17:45

DAVID WAS NOT supposed to fight Goliath. He was just the little shepherd boy delivering food. But when he saw Goliath blaspheming God, he simply knew he had to fight. No one believed in him—not his brothers, not the king—and his oldest brother was angry with him. He stood up anyway. He believed God's promise and had seen the power of God move before. He brought the most powerful weapon: almighty God.

TAKE HEART

Are you in a battle? If so, are you using the right weapon? The Bible says, "For though we live in the world, we do not wage war as the world does. The weapons we fight with are not the weapons of the world. On the contrary, they have divine power to demolish strongholds" (2 Cor. 10:3–4).

TAKE ACTION

Do you have a Goliath in your life? An addiction? A broken relationship? A fear? A regret? A crisis? Do you believe that God can deliver you? Are you trying to do it without God or too afraid to even try? Today is the day!

Day 27
BUT I REALLY MESSED UP

Then David sent messengers to get her. She came to him,
and he slept with her. (Now she was purifying herself from
her monthly uncleanness.) Then she went back home.
—2 Samuel 11:4

King David had an affair. And it only got worse from there: when he tried to cover it up, it led to murder. King David, in the lineage of Jesus, was an adulterer and murderer. I doubt many of us could check both of those boxes, and if we could (even in our thoughts), God is bigger.

Sometimes we look at our lives and think we are too far gone. We can never be redeemed. We've made bad choices for decades. Here's the truth: God is bigger than all of it. Of course, we must repent. We must own up to our sin and allow the Lord to heal our hearts and restore and redeem us. Only He can do that! But, boy, can He *do it*!

Take Heart

Have you messed up? Do you have a messy past? Present? Are you living a destructive lifestyle? No matter where you are right now, know this: it's not too late!

Take Action

Humble yourself. Repent and ask the Lord to forgive you. Ask for His grace to forgive yourself. And then move on in your anointing.

Day 28
RESURRECTED

*The LORD heard Elijah's cry, and the boy's
life returned to him, and he lived.*
—1 KINGS 17:22

THERE ARE SEVERAL instances in Scripture of death giving way to life, both literal and metaphorical. Of course, there is only one resurrected person who is *still alive*! However, the healing power of Jesus is as alive as ever, greater than we can even comprehend. If you ever doubt the healing, wonder-working power of God, simply put your hand on your chest and feel your heart beat. That is a miracle! Every single time. Or watch a cut heal or witness a broken bone mend. Your life and body are filled with countless miracles.

TAKE HEART

If the power that created and sustains you and has literally raised people from the dead is alive and in you today, then anything is possible!

TAKE ACTION

Is there a healing you have given up on? Or something you stopped crying out to God for? Is it time to resurrect that prayer? *Go for it!*

Day 29

GOD OF MIRACLES...AND
MIRACLES...AND MIRACLES

*The man of God asked, "Where did it fall?" When
he showed him the place, Elisha cut a stick and
threw it there, and made the iron float.*
—2 KINGS 6:6

WE DON'T OFTEN think of 2 Kings as full of miracles, but in
this book, God caused a widow's oil to keep flowing until
every jar was filled (4:2–6), raised a boy from the dead (4:20–35),
kept dangerous gourds cooked in a stew from harming anyone
(4:38–41), healed a man of leprosy (5:1–14), and, of course, made
iron float. This is the God we serve. He is a wonder-working,
miracle-making God. All the time.

I would suggest that miracles are constantly happening in
and around us. Whether the Lord is supernaturally covering
debts, raising the dead, cleansing poisoned food, healing diseases, or making iron float, it is amazing. And He still does
extraordinary things like that today.

TAKE HEART

If you saw or experienced God's miracle-working power, what
would change?

TAKE ACTION

Attend a healing service. Read some books about healing.
Watch some videos and testimonials about His healing power.
Challenge your beliefs, and challenge how you see the wonder-
working power of the risen Christ.

Day 30
PRIDE

Satan...incited David to take a census of Israel....Joab reported the number of the fighting men to David....But...the king's command was repulsive to him. This command was also evil in the sight of God; so he punished Israel. Then David said to God, "I have sinned greatly by doing this. Now, I beg you, take away the guilt of your servant. I have done a very foolish thing."
—1 Chronicles 21:1, 5–8

EVEN A GREAT king like David, a man after God's heart, with all his amazing experiences, can make mistakes. Sometimes we take credit for God's work. As a matter of fact, we do this all the time. We celebrate the illusion of the "self-made man," but there is no such thing. Shaping our lives is the work of God and God alone. (We often do a good job of messing it up.)

When David let pride slip in, the Lord brought correction. The Lord is a loving and jealous God. He will do whatever He has to do. When it comes to health, wellness, and healing, don't let pride slip in. God even gave you the brain you use to think about caring for yourself. He gave you a body to perform work and exercise.

TAKE HEART

When is the last time you thanked God for the body He gave you? For your beating heart? For putting breath in your lungs as you sleep?

TAKE ACTION

Identify an area of pride. Then repent.

DO YOU HAVE A HEART CONDITION?

*I know, my God, that you test the heart and are pleased
with integrity. All these things I have given willingly and
with honest intent. And now I have seen with joy how willingly your people who are here have given to you.*
—1 CHRONICLES 29:17

I USE A TEST called heart rate variability (HRV) in my office.
I love this test. The Scriptures often talk about the condition of the heart. Well, in some ways this test measures that.
It helps us see whether a person' s heart and nerve system can
adapt to the needs around them. The more adaptable, the
better the person's health.

The interesting aspect of this is that the way to improve
your heart variability is multifactorial. Many things influence
the health of your heart, including the food you eat, your fitness, exposure to toxins, and stress levels.

TAKE HEART

Guard your heart. How well are you monitoring the condition
of your heart?

TAKE ACTION

Get an HRV test done to see how you are adapting.

Day 32

FIRE FROM HEAVEN

*When Solomon finished praying, fire came down from heaven
and consumed the burnt offering and the sacrifices, and the
glory of the LORD filled the temple. The priests could not enter
the temple of the LORD because the glory of the LORD filled it.
When all the Israelites saw the fire coming down and the glory
of the LORD above the temple, they knelt on the pavement with
their faces to the ground, and they worshiped and gave thanks
to the LORD, saying, "He is good; his love endures forever."*
—2 CHRONICLES 7:1–3

CAN YOU IMAGINE being at this dedication event and, right
after the prayer, seeing fire from heaven consume the
offering and sacrifices? The Bible says after that, the presence
of the Lord was so thick that all anyone could do was lay on
the ground and say, "He is good; his love endures forever."

That really happened. And it will happen again. If you witnessed such a thing, how would it impact you?

TAKE HEART

Have you put yourself in positions to experience God's power?
Have you been seeking God's presence with reckless abandon?
When is the last time you got on your knees or on your face
and worshipped the Lord?

TAKE ACTION

Turn on some worship music, and get on your face before the
Lord. If you don't know what to say, just say, "You are good,
and Your love endures forever."

Day 33
THE NAYSAYERS

*Then the peoples around them set out to discourage the
people of Judah and make them afraid to go on building.*
—EZRA 4:4

WHEN YOU SET out to make bold moves in God-honoring
ways, make no mistake, you will meet resistance. This
resistance can come from well-intentioned men and women,
spiritual people, and at times even ourselves. Also, today's
culture is mostly anti-God. This is very important to understand because when you decide to live a God-honoring, holy,
righteous life abiding with God's laws, the world will tell you
that you're wrong, crazy, old-fashioned, etc. You must not
focus on that. Listen to God, not the enemy.

TAKE HEART

In what area or areas of your life have you let others' opinions
or the world discourage you? What areas of your lifestyle has
culture influenced in ungodly ways?

TAKE ACTION

Be bold. There is no need to apologize for living out the call
God has on your life.

Day 34
NO EXCUSES

When I heard these things, I sat down and wept. For some days I mourned and fasted and prayed before the God of heaven. Then I said: "LORD, the God of heaven...let your ear be attentive and your eyes open to hear the prayer your servant is praying before you day and night for your servants, the people of Israel. I confess the sins we Israelites, including myself and my father's family, have committed against you."
—NEHEMIAH 1:4–6

WE ALWAYS HEAR of new things happening. When we get such information, we can either take action or just ignore it. Often, when we learn of corruption, sin, and evil, we say someone should do something. Well, that someone might be *you*. When Nehemiah learned Jerusalem's wall had been broken down, he did something about it. He cried out to God, and then he led a campaign to rebuild the wall.

We often find excuses for why we can't take action: "I can't afford it"; "I don't have the time." The reality is that God provides *all* you need for the work He has for you. The enemy will always offer us excuses. But God always makes a way.

TAKE HEART

What has God placed in your heart that really impacts or moves you to action? What gives you holy delight?

TAKE ACTION

Do something—volunteer, find a church, join a gym, start a business. Just do *something*!

Day 35
FOR A TIME SUCH AS THIS

*When Esther's words were reported to Mordecai, he sent
back this answer: "Do not think that because you are in
the king's house you alone of all the Jews will escape. For
if you remain silent at this time, relief and deliverance for
the Jews will arise from another place, but you and your
father's family will perish. And who knows but that you
have come to your royal position for such a time as this?"*
—ESTHER 4:12–14

YOU HAVE LIKELY read this passage before. It can inspire,
embolden, encourage, or intimidate us. Here is a little
context: Esther was scared. She was not sure how her request
would be received. Even though she knew the right thing to do
for God's people, she was afraid to take a potentially unpopular
position. She was scared to go against the grain and stand out,
but she faced the fear and did it anyway. Thank God she did!

Following the will of God and living a godly life will not
be popular. Do it anyway. Speak up. Speak out. Do what God
says is right.

TAKE HEART

Do you find it hard to speak up and speak out against ungodly
things? Why? Do you think God approves?

TAKE ACTION

The next time you see something that goes against God, say
something. Speak up, even if it's just to a friend or family
member. Share God's perspective.

WILL YOU PASS THE TEST?

The LORD said to Satan, "Very well, then, everything he has is in your power, but on the man himself do not lay a finger."
—JOB 1:12

IF THE LORD allowed Satan to destroy everything you have in your life—family, finances, health, and friends—do you think you would lose your faith? Or when He searched your heart, would God see a person able to lose everything and keep his or her faith? This is Job. His incredible story is both heartbreaking and inspiring. Many people lose their faith or question God when bad things happen. They lose hope. Job's story shows us God alone is worthy of our trust. His ways are higher than ours. He is worthy if our worship, even when we do not like our circumstances.

TAKE HEART

Are there areas where you have suffered loss that you don't think God can redeem or restore? Don't lose hope. Remember, God's ways are higher than our ways (Isa. 55:8–9).

TAKE ACTION

Repent for lack of faith. Press back in to God, even in the face of insurmountable odds.

Day 37
ALL FOR NOTHING

*But you are plasterers of falsehood; you
are all physicians of no value.*
—JOB 13:4, MEV

THE POSSIBILITY THAT health care might cause net harm is
increasingly important given the sheer magnitude of the
modern health care enterprise. Serious review of these issues
will likely challenge assumptions about the value of many
current healthcare practices," wrote Dr. Charles Kilo and Dr.
Eric Larson.[1]

The results of studies that have looked at the harmful
effects of our current medical system are very concerning. It
is likely (I would say *certain*) that our medical system overall
causes more harm than help. Imagine if fire departments
caused more fires than they put out! That would seem odd,
yet our health-care "system," which costs us over four trillion
dollars per year, many times does more harm than good. This
should concern you and make you pause.

TAKE HEART

Why do you suppose our health-care system may result in
more harm than help?

TAKE ACTION

Many of us have simply trusted our doctors for so many years
that it can often feel overwhelming, or even scary, to make
changes. Ask yourself what you can do to avoid the limits,
risks, dangers, and expense of our current medical system.

Day 38
WHEN FRIENDS FAIL

*Then Job replied: "I have heard many things like these;
you are miserable comforters, all of you! Will your long-
winded speeches never end? What ails you that you keep
on arguing? I also could speak like you, if you were in
my place; I could make fine speeches against you and
shake my head at you. But my mouth would encourage
you; comfort from my lips would bring you relief."*
—JOB 16:1–5

JOB'S FRIENDS SHOWED up to "help" comfort him. But when things did not go as they hoped, they began to accuse him, saying untrue things and blaming him for the hardship he was facing.

Have you heard the saying "Misery loves company"? Be careful whom you let into your life, both in good times and bad. They may have good intentions, but not *God* intentions. God has the final word, just as He did with Job: "The LORD restored his fortunes and gave him twice as much as he had before." In fact, "the LORD blessed the latter part of Job's life more than the former part" (Job 42:10, 12).

TAKE HEART

Do you have friends who speak life and truth to you? Do you speak life and truth to them? Is God your ultimate friend?

TAKE ACTION

Read Job 38–42. God is God. You are not. Never, ever forget that.

PERVERTED

I have sinned and perverted what was
right, and it did not profit me.
—JOB 33:27, MEV

HERE ARE SOME heartbreaking statistics: 1 in 11 kids are on psychotropic medication;[1] almost 1 in 8 American adults have lifestyle-induced diabetes;[2] often-preventable health problems such as diabetes and heart disease ultimately lead to 7 in 10 deaths each year;[3] about 1 in 4 adults over age forty are on cholesterol drugs;[4] 1 in 6 kids are considered developmentally disabled,[5] which research suggests can stem from lifestyle and environmental factors; 1 in 5 preteens are obese;[6] almost 1 in 5 women are on antidepressants;[7] 2 in 5 Americans develop cancer;[8] and 1 in 5 people die from heart disease.[9]

This is not a good reflection of how God created our bodies to function. We have done a great job of *messing our bodies up*! Just like Adam and Eve in the Garden, we aren't satisfied with God's perfect design. We believe the enemy's lies that we need something more than what God has provided, so we take his offer. And our health suffers as a result.

TAKE HEART

When you read the statistics above, how does it make you feel? What do you think we should do?

TAKE ACTION

What needs to change in your life? Don't be satisfied with what the culture calls common.

Day 40

WHERE WERE YOU WHEN I CREATED IT ALL?

Where were you when I laid the earth's foundation? Tell me, if you understand.
—Job 38:4

I HAVE A PICTURE of an immune system attacking a cancer cell. I love looking at it because it reminds me how incredible the immune system God gave me is and how much is happening in my body without my knowledge. Amazing. God put wisdom in our bodies, equipping our immune systems to know how to find, destroy, and remove cancer cells. I love that; don't you?

TAKE HEART

Are you fearful of cancer? Do you spend more time worrying about cancer or thanking God for your amazing immune system?

TAKE ACTION

Our lifestyle choices impact cancer growth and destruction, especially when we eat lots of sugar. Consider your lifestyle. Is it beating or building cancer?

Day 41
WATER YOUR PLANTS!

He will be like a tree planted by the rivers of water,
that brings forth its fruit in its season; its leaf will not
wither, and whatever he does will prosper.
—PSALM 1:3, MEV

WHAT DO YOUR plants look like around the house? Are the leaves wilting or brown? If so, you may do a couple of things. You may need to give them some water, sunshine, or plant food. Assuming they are not too far gone, the plants will recover. The plants will heal. Now, I doubt you would call the news station to report a miraculous resurrection. You know that if the plant gets what it needs, it will heal.

It is the same with your body. Give it what it needs; let God do the rest. Some of us have more faith in a plant's ability to heal than we do in our own body's!

TAKE HEART

Do you have more faith in a plant's ability to heal than in your own body's? Why or why not?

TAKE ACTION

Today, add some water, sunshine, and nutrition to your day! Expect a miracle!

Day 42
WHO IS YOUR SHEPHERD?

*The LORD is my shepherd; I shall not want. He makes me lie
down in green pastures; He leads me beside still waters.
He restores my soul; He leads me in paths of righteousness for His name's sake. Even though I walk through the
valley of the shadow of death, I will fear no evil; for You
are with me; Your rod and Your staff, they comfort me.*
—PSALM 23:1–4, MEV

YOU CAN ALLOW anything to be your shepherd. So I want
to ask, What is shepherding your heart? Instagram? Facebook? Netflix? Sex? Drugs? Pornography? Money? Booze?
Food?

It is critical that we choose a good shepherd. Jesus is the
Good Shepherd (John 10:11, 14). And I know this may be hard
to believe in today's selfie culture, but He loves you more than
you love yourself.

TAKE HEART

Consider how you are spending your time and whom you're
spending it with. Jesus wants our whole hearts.

TAKE ACTION

If you believe you're letting social or other types of media
lead you, pray about deleting social media apps or putting
your television in a closet and spending a season fasting or
detoxing from those influences. Pray first for the Lord to
reveal to you what has your heart.

CREATE IN ME A CLEAN HEART, O LORD!

Have mercy on me, O God, according to your unfailing love; according to your great compassion blot out my transgressions. Wash away all my iniquity and cleanse me from my sin....Cleanse me with hyssop, and I will be clean; wash me, and I will be whiter than snow....Create in me a pure heart, O God, and renew a steadfast spirit within me.
—PSALM 51:1–2, 7, 10

ONE OF THE leading causes of death is heart disease. This is true physically and spiritually. When David asked the Lord to search and clean his heart, he wasn't asking for a good car wash or sprinkling. It was a lot more like a supernatural heart transplant. Caring for our hearts begins first in the spiritual realm and then the physical. Many physicians say a primary risk factor for heart disease is stress. Stress often occurs when we are outside the plans and purposes of God.

TAKE HEART

Is your lifestyle stressing your heart?

TAKE ACTION

Ask the Lord to search and cleanse your heart. Ask Him to show you one or two areas you need to clean up. Maybe it's forgiveness, or maybe it's Twinkies.

Day 44
BONES HEAL

Make me to hear joy and gladness, that the
bones that You have broken may rejoice.
—PSALM 51:8, MEV

THE HEALING OF a broken bone is fascinating! The bone totally remodels and heals itself. How does it know how to do this? The cast does not heal the break. The power God put in our bodies does. Amazing! It is incredible to think God made it possible for a broken bone to reknit itself together and be as strong as it was before.[1]

TAKE HEART

Why do we take bones healing for granted? Why do we expect bones to heal but think healing from heart disease, cancer, or diabetes is too difficult?

TAKE ACTION

Consider how incredible it is that a cut heals. Be inspired and encouraged by the wonder-working power of God!

Day 45
THE HEART OF THE MATTER

Create in me a clean heart, O God, and
renew a right spirit within me.
—PSALM 51:10, MEV

ACCORDING TO DR. Dean Ornish, "Studies have shown
that changing lifestyle could prevent at least 90% of all
heart disease. Thus, the disease that accounts for more pre-
mature deaths and costs Americans more than any other illness is almost completely preventable and even reversible,
simply by changing lifestyle."[1]

Heart disease is a top killer in the United States, yet it is
almost entirely preventable. Many doctors treat it by pre-
scribing medications without addressing the person's actual
lifestyle. More of us are taking medications for heart disease
than ever before, yet the rate of heart disease continues to
rise.[2] Scripture talks a lot about the condition of our hearts.
Are you taking good care of yours?

TAKE HEART

Are you surprised that heart disease is preventable? Do you
know the things you can do to care for your cardiovascular
system?

TAKE ACTION

Look up Dr. Dean Ornish and view some of his basic suggestions for cardiovascular health.

THEY ARE CORRUPT

The fool says in his heart, "There is no God." They are corrupt, and their ways are vile....God looks down from heaven...to see if there are...any who seek God. Everyone has turned away, all have become corrupt; there is no one who does good, not even one.
—PSALM 53:1–3

D O YOU THINK there is corruption in the world? Gallup recently did a poll asking how much people trust different businesses. Does it surprise you that the three least-trusted industries are (1) pharmaceuticals, (2) government, and (3) health care? And this poll was done in 2019—*before* the COVID-19 pandemic.[1]

As believers, it is crucial we have discernment. The reality is, there are corrupt businesses and people who do not have God or your best interests in mind. They are built on greed and manipulation. Sometimes Jesus had to tip the tables!

TAKE HEART

Do you struggle to trust certain industries? Or do you trust them more than God? When you consider how much influence we have allowed the least-trusted industries to have in our lives, you can see the problem we have.

TAKE ACTION

Do your part. Stay educated. Don't just go along with everything because someone told you to. Do not be deceived. Be on guard. Not everything is as it appears.

Day 47
WHEN YOUR FLESH FAILS

My flesh and my heart may fail, but God is the
strength of my heart and my portion forever.
—PSALM 73:26

WE ARE ALL going to die. Sorry for the buzzkill, but it is critical that we remember this fact. We cannot let our lives become idols. Self-preservation is the ultimate Holy Spirit quencher. Your flesh will eventually fail. You will die. Are you living in full awareness of that reality?

And let me remind you that eternity is a lot longer than our time here on earth. Are you storing up treasures in heaven or building a temporary empire on earth? I have heard it said this way: Are you decorating your hotel room or furnishing your eternal home?

TAKE HEART

Do you fear death? If not, why? If so, how does that affect your daily choices?

TAKE ACTION

If you had one year to live, what would you change and why? Don't just make a mental list. Write it down. What would God think of your list? Do you need to make any lifestyle changes?

Day 48

A BLAMELESS WALK

*I will be careful to lead a blameless life—when will you
come to me? I will conduct the affairs of my house with
a blameless heart. I will not look with approval on anything that is vile. I hate what faithless people do; I will
have no part in it. The perverse of heart shall be far
from me; I will have nothing to do with what is evil.*
—PSALM 101:2–4

WE OFTEN LIKE to straddle the fence. Dietrich Bonhoeffer
wrote about a concept called "cheap grace" that tries to
let us off the hook without us really repenting and owning
up to our sinful or fleshly lifestyles.[1] God does not take luke-
warm believers lightly. He does not do well with halfway hypocrites. Yes, He gives us "grace upon grace" (John 1:16, MEV),
but we need to press into a righteous life in all areas. This is
not possible in our own power.

TAKE HEART

God is with you and for you. He wants what is best for you—
which is Him and His ways. How do you see sin? How do you
think Jesus views it?

TAKE ACTION

Where is there wickedness around you? Where is there wickedness in your heart? Repent and surrender it to God.

THIS IS YOUR BRAIN ON SUGAR

*...who satisfies your mouth with good things, so
that your youth is renewed like the eagle's.*
—Psalm 103:5, mev

THERE IS AN image of two scans that show the brain's response to sugar versus cocaine. It's easy to see how similar the reactions are. There is a reason we crave certain foods. Our brains literally respond to sugar more strongly than they do to cocaine! This is why we can eat a whole bag of Doritos and not almonds. We are programmed to crave and become addicted to these foods.[1] We need to use the motto "Let the buyer beware" when shopping for foods. We can become unknowingly addicted to the chemicals in food and suffer accordingly.

TAKE HEART

Do you eat a lot of processed food? Sugar? Artificial colors? Have you considered a detox?

TAKE ACTION

Learn to read labels and ingredients. If there are lots of ingredients you can't pronounce, they probably are not good for you. Remember, you are what you eat.

Day 50
ARE YOU THANKFUL?

*Praise the LORD. Give thanks to the LORD, for
he is good; his love endures forever.*
—PSALM 106:1

MANY HEALTH-CARE PROVIDERS will tell you that thankfulness or gratitude is critical to maintaining your health, both physical and mental.[1] We often focus on what we don't have (covet), and this discontent can drive us into anxiety, depression, and the like. I am always inspired by stories of people who have suffered great tragedy yet are grateful even in the midst of those hardships. Gratitude is a choice. You can choose to be thankful.

TAKE HEART

Are you grateful? Do people who know you think you are a thankful person?

TAKE ACTION

List one hundred things you are grateful for. You might include your sight and other senses, a beating heart, a full tummy, your kids, your spouse, and so on.

Day 51

THE LORD'S PROTECTION

The Lord shall protect you from all evil;
He shall preserve your soul.
—Psalm 121:7, mev

W<small>E NEED THE</small> Lord's protection, and we need to use wisdom to avoid known and unknown dangers. An Environmental Protection Agency (EPA) inventory lists over 86,000 chemicals (not including pesticides and food additives) used in today's commercial products.[1] But as late as 2016, the EPA had tested only a tiny percentage[2] and banned just nine of those chemicals.[3]

Statistics like these are almost unbelievable. It can be frustrating when we learn a product or food we have been using for years is actually dangerous. These products can lead to things like asthma, eczema, allergies, and even cancer if we are exposed long-term. In today's world, we need to be savvy consumers. We can't often trust the marketing or many of the agencies we are told to trust.

TAKE HEART

We need to understand that the chemicals, foods, words, TV, and social media we allow into our lives have effects, both good and bad. We all fall short of God's glory, but that is not an excuse to make poor or ignorant choices. We need to do our part.

TAKE ACTION

Go to EWG.org and learn more about the products you are using in your home. You may be shocked.

Day 52

EACH OF US IS UNIQUE

You created my inmost being; you knit me
together in my mother's womb.
—PSALM 139:13

EMBRYOS DEVELOP FINGERPRINTS three months after conception. This is important to note, especially as people debate about life and whether a fetus is unique. Well, over the billions of people who have existed since God created mankind, no two fingerprints have ever been the same. God says you are one of a kind. You are designed for a specific purpose. Even if someone says you don't matter or that you are a mistake or unwanted, you are wanted by God—always.

TAKE HEART

You have always mattered. Do you feel loved by God? Do you spend time with the One who made your fingerprints?

TAKE ACTION

Take a few minutes to thank God for all the things He does for you. When is the last time you thanked Him for your fingerprints (which actually have a purpose)?

HE KNOWS EACH OF US BY NAME

I will praise you, for You made me with fear and wonder;
marvelous are Your works, and You know me completely.
—PSALM 139:14, MEV

SOMETIMES EXTRAORDINARY CIRCUMSTANCES give us a glimpse into just how amazing and complex the bodies God gave us are. Masha and Dasha, born in Russia in the 1950s, were conjoined twins who shared all major systems of the body (blood, digestive, lymph, and endocrine) but had their own spines and nerve systems. Here is what is fascinating: Because of their separate nervous systems, one would get the flu, and the other wouldn't! They shared the same blood, but one would get measles, and the other would not. This shows us the incredible complexity of our bodies and the importance of our nerve systems.

TAKE HEART

After God made mankind, He said it was very good. Never forget whose image you are made in.

TAKE ACTION

What is one area of health or your body that fascinates you?

Day 54

HE HUNG THE MOON!

*He determines the number of the stars
and calls them each by name.*
—Psalm 147:4

Scientists estimate that there are one hundred trillion atoms in a human cell. And there are anywhere from thirty-seven trillion to one hundred trillion cells in the human body! Just do this math. Not only that, but each of these cells is performing countless processes per second. And you think about none of them. In His wisdom the same God who hung the stars and spins the earth created *you* and keeps you functioning. It is an absolutely mind-boggling fact that should leave you in awe!

Take Heart

What is one hundred trillion times one hundred trillion? It is 10,000,000,000,000,000,000,000,000,000. That's what your body is doing right now with zero thought on your end! Your heart beats, your lungs breathe, your eyes see, and your ears hear, just as God created them to.

Take Action

Stop and give thanks for the body God gave you.

Day 55
MAKE TIME

My son, if you will receive my words, and
hide my commandments within you...
—Proverbs 2:1, MEV

IF I HAD a nickel for every time a patient has told me he doesn't have time to care for his body, I would be a very wealthy man. We have time for the things we value. We adults average watching three and a half hours of TV a day. I think we have time for some motion. With some of the newer exercise techniques, such as high-intensity interval training (HIIT), we can do a lot in a short amount of time.

TAKE HEART

Have you ever made the excuse that you're too busy to care for your body? Are you still making this excuse? What would it take to get you moving more?

TAKE ACTION

When we were young children, we often complained and pouted when our parents made us do things we didn't want to do. Some of us have taken up that habit as adults! Don't act like a baby.

Day 56
TRUST THE LORD

*Trust in the LORD with all your heart and lean not on
your own understanding; in all your ways submit
to him, and he will make your paths straight.*
—PROVERBS 3:5–6

GOD IS NOT dumb. He didn't create our bodies to express
symptoms to torture us. They are part of His divine
design. It is OK to have symptoms and let your body heal.
Not every symptom needs a pill, shot, oil, or label. Not every
fever needs to be lowered, and not every cough needs to be
suppressed. It is OK to just let symptoms run their course.
Some symptoms don't need to be treated. They are often
signs that the healing is happening! Prescription drugs are
often so heavily marketed here in the United States that we
almost subconsciously reach for something to relieve or treat
symptoms because we think they need to be masked. But not
feeling a symptom doesn't mean the problem has gone away,
and sometimes masking the issue only makes it worse.

TAKE HEART

Do you tend to reach for something to treat your symptoms
the moment you begin to experience them? Why? How does
knowing the symptom may actually be part of the cure affect
your perspective?

TAKE ACTION

Next time you get the sniffles, challenge yourself to let yourself heal without taking something.

Day 57
ARE YOU WISE?

*Blessed are those who find wisdom, those who
gain understanding, for she is more profitable than
silver and yields better returns than gold.*
—Proverbs 3:13–14

I KNOW MANY SMART people, but I do not know many *wise*
people. Solomon asked for wisdom so he could be a blessing
to others (1 Kings 3:9). That is why God honored his request.

TAKE HEART

Would you consider yourself wise? Why or why not?
Experience is not wisdom. It does not come through a Google
search. Wisdom is a gift from God, and we must be intentional about seeking it. James 1:5 says, "If any of you lacks
wisdom, you should ask God, who gives generously to all
without finding fault, and it will be given to you." If you consider yourself wise, how are you using your wisdom for the
good of others?

TAKE ACTION

Have you ever prayed for wisdom? Think of a time the Lord
gave you wisdom. Are you stewarding it well? In what areas
would you like to have more wisdom?

Day 58
DISCIPLINE IS FREEDOM

*Whoever heeds discipline shows the way to life, but
whoever ignores correction leads others astray.*
—PROVERBS 10:17

THE WORD *DISCIPLINE* has a mostly negative connotation
in today's culture. We think of discipline as hard, restrictive, and a loss of choice. But Solomon tells us it is "the way to life." And he goes a step further to say if we are undisciplined, it will lead others astray! The last thing any of us would want to do is cause another to stumble or be led astray by our lack of discipline.

TAKE HEART

Do you consider yourself disciplined? Think about your life. Are you a slave in any area: to food, alcohol, social media, sex? In what areas do you need to be disciplined?

TAKE ACTION

Pick an area and take action for at least thirty days. You might choose to read the Bible for thirty minutes each day, change your eating habits, or log off social media. You can do this, "for the Spirit God gave us does not make us timid, but gives us power, love and self-discipline" (2 Tim. 1:7).

DEAD WRONG

There is a way that appears to be right, but
in the end it leads to death.
—PROVERBS 14:12

OFTENTIMES OUR CHOICES have unintended consequences. Maybe something sounded like a good idea at the time, but looking back, it wasn't. Think of the countless medications that were once celebrated as the next great medical wonder but were later pulled from the market after harming or killing thousands of people. The "side effects" were sometimes fatal. In the same way, culture, corporations, government, and social media may have an agenda that is not of God (sin) and will lead to death.

TAKE HEART

Can you think of a time or two when you saw this principle in action?

TAKE ACTION

What is an area where you are currently trusting in mankind or society more than God? Identify it, repent, and pray that you will not return to that way of thinking. Choose life, not death!

THERE IS A WAY THAT SEEMS RIGHT

*There is a way that appears to be right, but
in the end it leads to death.*
—PROVERBS 14:12

THIS MAY SHOCK you. Here is a list of only *some* of the potential long-term effects of children taking antibiotics before their first birthday: significant increased risk of Crohn's, juvenile arthritis, major infections, asthma, and obesity (by up to 15 percent). Antibiotics destroy the gut biome.[1] They are not vitamins; they are anti-bio. *Bio* means "life." Anything that is anti-life we should pause on. This is one of many areas of modern medicine that we need to reconsider.

TAKE HEART

Do you think antibiotics are overprescribed? Do you think you need them to heal?

TAKE ACTION

Research some natural approaches to viral and bacterial infections. God gave you a couple of amazing ones that are built in: fevers and immune systems. Thank God for fevers and vomit!

Day 61
POWER OF WORDS

A healing tongue is a tree of life, but a
deceitful one crushes the spirit.
—PROVERBS 15:4, TLV

YOU HAVE LIKELY heard that "the tongue has the power of life and death" (Prov. 18:21). The words we say to others and our own self-talk are literally bringing life or death. I've read reports of a doctor or someone in authority giving a person a prognosis such as, "You have six months to live," and the person dying almost to the day. In some instances it was later discovered that the person didn't even have the disease.[1] But the power of those words and the person's faith in the authority figure were so strong, it actually caused them to die.

TAKE HEART

Do you believe this? How is your self-talk? Have you ever had a diagnosis spoken into your life (due to a family history of diabetes, cancer, high blood pressure, or the like)? Did you receive it?

TAKE ACTION

While negative words bring death, the opposite is true too. The right words bring life, healing, and truth. Take inventory of the talk that you surround yourself with and that you speak to yourself. Be intentional about speaking life and surrounding yourself with life-giving words!

Day 62
LOVE TO EAT?

*Better a small serving of vegetables with love
than a fattened calf with hatred.*
—Proverbs 15:17

SOME PEOPLE HATE eating in a healthy way so much so that the attitude and stress it causes outweigh the positives of the food. Yet when we make lifestyle changes, we do it as a form of worship unto the Lord, not with resentment or out of obligation. Now, of course, this is a journey, as it involves changing our habits and reframing our food choices. But above all, remember to be thankful for what you are eating. Also, be mindful of when and where you are eating. Ideally our meals should not be consumed in a stressed, rushed atmosphere. Eating in a relaxed environment actually helps our digestion.

TAKE HEART

Do you enjoy eating well, or do you love junk food? What do you think God thinks about this?

TAKE ACTION

Before your next meal, no matter what it is, pause and reflect before you partake. Give thanks to God.

Day 63
MOVE IT OR LOSE IT

The way of the slothful man is as a hedge of thorns,
but the way of the righteous is made plain.
—Proverbs 15:19, mev

SITTING IS THE new smoking. Recent studies have shown that our sedentary lifestyles (sitting at our desks, for example) are harder on our health than smoking.[1] We sit and watch TV, we sit in cars, we sit at work, and so on—and all this sitting is impacting our health. Posture affects everything from pain to breathing to even hormones. It is critical that we move. God designed us to move. "Move it or lose it," as the adage goes. Jesus was active; are you?

Take Heart

Motion is life. Do you value movement? How much movement are you getting? Twenty to thirty minutes three to five times a week is ideal.

Take Action

Be honest with yourself. Reflect on your daily schedule. Are you making time for movement? You likely choose not to smoke because of the health concerns. Choose to move for the same reasons.

Day 64
TRUST GOD'S DESIGN

There is a way that seems right to a man,
but its end is the way of death.
—PROVERBS 16:25, MEV

WHEN YOU PUT all the substances in God-made breast milk against man-made baby formula, you can really see the contrast of God's way versus man's. There are over two hundred different ingredients in moms' milk compared to about forty-six in formula.[1]

We often get so enamored by man's plans that we actually give them more credit than we do God's plans. It never works out well for us in the long run. You can't rob Peter to pay Paul.

TAKE HEART

In what other areas have humans attempted to improve on God's design? How has that worked out?

TAKE ACTION

Challenge yourself to consider whether you have made idols out of any areas, especially relating to health care. Do you have more faith in pills, vaccines, or testing than you do the God who created you? If anything like this has become an idol for you, repent and put your confidence in the Lord your Maker.

HOPELESS?

A person's spirit sustains him through sickness—
but who can bear a crushed spirit?
—PROVERBS 18:14, NET

HAVE YOU KNOWN someone who was given a negative diagnosis or had something tragic happen and just seemed to give up? On the other hand, have you met someone who seems to have such a resilient spirit that no matter what life throws at her, she faces it with hope? The spirit the Lord puts in us allows us to be fearless and full of hope. As a matter of fact, I would suggest that hope is evidence that we are filled with the Holy Spirit.

TAKE HEART

Are you familiar with the baptism of the Holy Spirit? Can you recall an experience or experiences where you felt the tangible presence of the Lord? If not, there is a great opportunity here for you to seek the baptism in the Holy Spirit. Theologian A. W. Tozer has some incredible writings on this, including *How to Be Filled With the Holy Spirit.*

TAKE ACTION

Find a church, pastor, or friend who is willing to lead you in being baptized in the Holy Spirit. If this concept is new to you, I implore you to read the Book of Acts, particularly Acts 2.

TOO MUCH OF A GOOD THING

Whoever loves pleasure will become poor; whoever loves wine and olive oil will never be rich.
—PROVERBS 21:17

WE LIVE IN a culture of quick fixes: do whatever feels good and gives good vibes. When hedonism is the siren call, wisdom like we see in this verse from Proverbs can almost seem offensive. Aren't we supposed to follow our passions and do what we love?

As believers, our first love is Christ. Anything that gets in the way of that in our hearts is idolatry and/or sin leading to death. It may feel good in the moment, but it leads to destruction.

TAKE HEART

Do you have some things in your life that you love, that bring you pleasure, but are not godly or righteous?

TAKE ACTION

Remember your first love, and return to Him. Nothing can fill that hole in your heart other than Jesus.

Day 67
CAN YOU SEE?

Where there is no vision, the people perish.
—PROVERBS 29:18, MEV

THE CORNEA IS the only part of the body with no blood supply. It gets its oxygen directly from the air. Today's scripture says that those with lack of vision will perish, or have no life. I think the unique aspect of the human cornea is a reminder of this. Physically, we need to keep our eyes (vision) open to keep getting oxygen to them or they will die. Spiritually, we need to do the same thing. Don't you just love how God ties these together?

TAKE HEART

Do you have a vision for your life? Have you talked to Jesus about it?

TAKE ACTION

If you don't feel like you have a God-given purpose or vision for your life, I know He would love to talk to you about it. Take some time. Read His Word. Pray for Him to show you!

Day 68
ARE YOU CHASING THE WIND?

I denied myself nothing my eyes desired; I refused my heart no
pleasure. My heart took delight in all my labor, and this was
the reward....Yet when I surveyed all that my hands had done
and what I had toiled to achieve, everything was meaningless,
a chasing after the wind; nothing was gained under the sun.
—ECCLESIASTES 2:10–11

SOLOMON HAD AND did it all—money, women, material
things, fame. You name it, he had it. Yet how did he sum it
all up? It was like chasing the wind. It all added up to nothing.

So many of us fall into the trap of wanting just a little more.
We think, "When I have _____, I will be happy. When I
earn more, I will help others and be more generous." The
sad fact is that it never really works that way. Sometimes it
feels that way briefly. We get the new car, new house, or new
T-shirt, and we feel good. But it fades. Solomon's warning and
wisdom attempt to save us from chasing the wind.

TAKE HEART

Have you been tempted to keep up with the Joneses or build
your own empire? What do you think Solomon would say?

TAKE ACTION

Do you need to get rid of anything in your life? Are there
things you strive for or are too attached to? What is one thing
you can let go of? Do it.

AS A TWIG IS BENT, SO GROWS THE TREE

Consider the work of God: Who is able to make straight what He has made crooked?
—ECCLESIASTES 7:13, MEV

A S A CHIROPRACTOR I see posture issues and spine X-rays on a daily basis. With all our texting, computer use, sedentary lifestyles, and poor posture, we are causing lots of posture and spinal problems that affect our health in a variety of ways. We brush our teeth two or three times a day, but spinal hygiene is even more important!

TAKE HEART

Do you have good posture? Do you try to sit upright? Are you careful when on your phone or computer? Do you monitor your sleep position? Is your posture hurting you?

TAKE ACTION

Look in the mirror. How is your posture? Are you standing straight? Now look at it from the side. Is your head forward? Are your shoulders humped? Get a postural stretch routine.[1] It just might change your life!

Day 70
LOVE LETTER

How beautiful you are, my darling! Oh, how
beautiful! Your eyes are doves.
—SONG OF SONGS 1:15

THERE ARE SEVERAL interpretations and many commentaries about what Song of Songs means, but I think anyone who reads this short book will be captivated by the intensity of the language and descriptions it provides. It's almost shocking and could make us a little uncomfortable. At times, it almost makes us blush. But it's all about love—God's love for us and ours for Him, God's love for His church and His church's for Him, and our love for others and others for us.

Sometimes we can get numb or stuck in a rut in our relationships even when things are good. Love is intense. Love is passionate. Love is powerful.

TAKE HEART

Do you remember the first time you were falling in love? What did it feel like?

TAKE ACTION

Write a love letter to a spouse, to a friend, or to God. Just pour out your heart.

HAVE WE MADE MODERN MEDICINE AN IDOL?

*Their land is full of idols; they bow down to the work
of their hands, to what their fingers have made.*
—ISAIAH 2:8

THE SAD REALITY is that the United States is the most medicated nation on earth. We are one of only two countries in the world that allow drug companies to advertise to people. There is "a pill for every ill." But the problem is that this has not worked. We are not a healthier people. And even sadder is that we are just as sick inside the church as outside the church. We have become "like the world," even though we are called to be a set-apart people.

TAKE HEART

Does it concern you how medicated we have become, especially our children? Do you think there is a better way?

TAKE ACTION

A majority of health concerns and symptoms are lifestyle related. Review your lifestyle. Do you need some help to get your health care or self-care back on track?

Day 72

POWER OF PRAYER

*Then the word of the LORD came to Isaiah: "Go and
tell Hezekiah, 'This is what the LORD, the God of your
father David, says: I have heard your prayer and seen
your tears; I will add fifteen years to your life.'"*
—ISAIAH 38:4–5

T HIS IS AN amazing story. Hezekiah was given a diagnosis of
certain death directly from the Lord through the prophet
Isaiah. Hezekiah immediately prayed, and the Bible says the
Lord heard his prayer and added fifteen years to his life.

There are many layers and metaphors to the story, but
consider this question: When you get bad news (in this case,
impending death), what is your first response? The lesson here
is that we should pray immediately, directly to God. And we
should expect a response much like the one Hezekiah received.
God's answer was personal (Scripture says He heard the prayer)
and specific (the Lord added years to his life). When we seek
the Lord, we can expect Him to hear us and respond with a
specific answer for our needs.

TAKE HEART

What do you think of Hezekiah's story? Do you think things
like this still happen today? Why or why not?

TAKE ACTION

Challenge yourself to make direct prayer your first response
to things that seem impossible, and watch what God does.
Expect God to move!

Day 73

JESUS LOVES YOU AT THE CELLULAR LEVEL!

Lift up your eyes and look to the heavens: Who created all these? He who brings out the starry host one by one and calls forth each of them by name. Because of his great power and mighty strength, not one of them is missing.
—ISAIAH 40:26

THERE IS A picture of one small part of one human immune cell, and it is mind blowing.[1] Now, consider this: in all of history from the beginning of time, mankind has never created a single cell. We cannot create life. Only God does that. Yet in the minute or two it took to read this, the power God put in your body has made *thousands* of cells! It is good to be in awe of God.

TAKE HEART

Why do people try to take credit for God's work? What does the Bible say about pride?

TAKE ACTION

Really consider the magnificence of the creation that is *you*. Meditate on the gift and miracle of life!

Day 74

HE IS A GENERATIONAL GOD

*Those from among you shall rebuild the old waste
places; you shall raise up the foundations of many generations; and you shall be called, the Repairer of the
Breach, the Restorer of Paths in which to Dwell.*
—ISAIAH 58:12, MEV

HAVE YOU EVER heard of Pottenger's cats? It is a fascinating study of generational health. The researcher fed
some cats food that was cooked (which lowered the nutrient
quality), and every subsequent generation became sicker and
sicker until they were not even able to reproduce.[1]

Your health affects not only you but also your future generations. And your health has been affected by those before you.
The Bible discusses generational blessings and curses, and the
same applies to our health.

TAKE HEART

Are you thinking generationally about your health? What lifestyles from past generations do you need to break?

TAKE ACTION

Look at your family history. Has it set you up for success? Do
you need to break some strongholds and change some habits
for your future?

WE NEED JESUS

*All of us have become like one who is unclean, and all
our righteous acts are like filthy rags; we all shrivel up
like a leaf, and like the wind our sins sweep us away.*
—ISAIAH 64:6

SOMETIMES WE JUSTIFY our unhealthy choices by saying we
make them only "once in a while." And of course that is
better than all the time, but it still has some long-term effects.
The reason is that the foods we eat become the body we have
tomorrow. It is important to realize that if we eat something
like a Twinkie, which is cooked with trans fats, its ingredients become integrated into our cells and take months to be
turned over in our bodies. But it is difficult to resist unhealthy
choices on our own. We need Jesus and the empowering of
the Holy Spirit.

TAKE HEART

Our bodies are constantly regenerating, but they use the
materials we give them. Are you giving your body good material to build with?

TAKE ACTION

What is your nutritional vice? What is one bad food habit you
would like to change? See if you can find a healthier alterna-
tive. For example, if you drink too much soda, maybe trying
carbonated water will help you avoid it.

MOTHER'S MILK

For you will nurse and be satisfied at her comforting breasts; you will drink deeply and delight in her overflowing abundance.
— ISAIAH 66:11

I REMEMBER READING ABOUT an experiment where researchers took petri dishes with bacteria in them and placed a drop of breast milk in the middle of each. It was amazing to see photos of how the breast milk killed the bacteria. It can kill viruses too.[1] Isn't it incredible what mother's milk created by God is capable of doing? Formula doesn't do that. God's design is the best design.

TAKE HEART

Studies done on the benefits of breast milk have shown unbelievable results, including increased IQ! What fascinates you about this?

TAKE ACTION

If the culture says something about health that goes against God's design, I would give it serious pause. Although there are circumstances that may prevent a woman from being able to breastfeed, we should contend for the benefits of breastfeeding.

Day 77
YOU ARE NOT ALONE

Before I formed you in the womb I knew you, before you were born I set you apart; I appointed you as a prophet to the nations.
—JEREMIAH 1:5

SOMETIMES TO MOVE forward, we have to go back to the beginning. God knows you really, really well! He knew you before you were even in your mother's womb. Think about that fact. He conceived you before you were conceived. Amazing! So if you struggle with feelings of worth, value, identity, or loneliness, remember this: the Creator of the universe, the heavens and the earth, created *you*, specifically!

TAKE HEART

Do you ever struggle to believe how much God loves you? Have you ever thought about how specific He was when He created you?

TAKE ACTION

Journal to God or say a prayer thanking Him for creating you. Thank Him for all the unique and special things about you!

Day 78
BEFORE YOU WERE EVEN BORN

Before I formed you in the womb I knew you, before you were born I set you apart; I appointed you as a prophet to the nations.
—JEREMIAH 1:5

A RELATIVELY NEW AREA of science is called epigenetics. *Epi-* means "upon" or "before." This is where we learn that the environment our genes are in is much more important than the genes themselves.

This is great news. Our genes are not our destiny. They play a role in our health outcomes, but our lifestyles play a much larger part. Research has shown that a majority of diseases are *not* genetic; they result from the environment we put our genes in.

TAKE HEART

Does this information surprise you? Encourage you? Convict you? What areas do you need to improve in?

TAKE ACTION

Rate your lifestyle on a scale of 1 to 10. Make a commitment to move the needle up the scale!

CHOOSE THE THINGS OF GOD

"This is your lot, the portion I have decreed for you,"
declares the LORD, "because you have
forgotten me and trusted in false gods."
—JEREMIAH 13:25

WE ARE OVERFED and undernourished. Think about that. What incredible times we live in. We are literally stuffing ourselves with junk and wondering why we are sick. If you filled your car with Coca-Cola and it didn't run, you would not be surprised. So why be surprised when filling your body with it (or other processed foods) affects your health?

You could also say we are overfed and undernourished with Scripture. We have more access than ever before, but we seem to be drifting further than ever away.

TAKE HEART

Why do you think we have become so addicted to processed foods and sugary food and drinks? What do you struggle with? Have you taken this struggle to the Lord?

TAKE ACTION

If it grew on a plant, eat it. If it is made in a manufacturing plant, don't.

DO NOT FEAR

I called on your name, LORD, from the depths of the pit. You heard my plea: "Do not close your ears to my cry for relief." You came near when I called you, and you said, "Do not fear."
—LAMENTATIONS 3:55–57

I HAVE HEARD IT preached that there are 365 "fear nots" in the Bible, one for each day of the year.[1] Whether or not this is accurate, the Bible clearly addresses the topic of fear again and again, and I don't think that is an accident. We need to be reminded that we are to fear one thing: God. All other things we fear expose our lack of faith. Do you fear dying? Why? Do you have fears concerning your finances? Do you fear what others say or think?

Two of the most common mental health issues in the United States are anxiety disorders and depression. Americans consume endless medications in an attempt to mask the pain. Addressing our fears or lack of faith could help with this struggle.

TAKE HEART

What are you afraid of? Why? Ask yourself that again: Why? What do you think God would say to you? He tells us again and again to *fear not*.

TAKE ACTION

Choose one thing you have some fear about. Pray, and then take a step to let go of that fear.

Day 81
A NEW HEART, STOMACH, AND LIVER

*I will give them an undivided heart and put a new
spirit in them; I will remove from them their heart
of stone and give them a heart of flesh.*
—EZEKIEL 11:19

RESEARCH HAS SHOWN how our bodies are always regenerating. For example, the blood is new every four months, the skin every month, the liver every seven to ten months, and the stomach lining about every five days! Incredible.

Isn't it fascinating how God created our bodies to regenerate and heal? Every year that goes by, we learn more and more about how amazing and resilient the body He created is. Let this encourage you and blow your mind.

TAKE HEART

Does knowing the body repairs and regenerates surprise you? Does it inspire and encourage you?

TAKE ACTION

Spend a few minutes thanking God for the amazing gift He gave you—your body—that He created in His likeness and image.

DRY BONES

Then he said to me, "Prophesy to these bones and say to them,
'...I will make breath enter you, and you will come to life....'" So
I prophesied as I was commanded. And as I was prophesying,
there was...a rattling sound, and the bones came together...and
tendons and flesh appeared on them and skin covered them....
Then he said to me, "Prophesy to the breath...that they may live."
So I prophesied as he commanded me, and breath entered
them; they came to life and stood up on their feet—a vast army.
—EZEKIEL 37:4–10

THIS ACCOUNT IN Ezekiel 37 is incredible. The prophet is placed in a valley full of dry bones, and the Lord empowers him to literally speak life into them. Can you imagine witnessing this? Well, in some sense you do. Your body is constantly rebuilding and repairing itself; even your bones are always rebuilding and regenerating. It's an incredible, miraculous marvel. Yet we often act (and feel) like we are too far gone, like the best is behind us, like it's too late for us and we could never heal or recover.

Well, I know of a valley filled with people who were so dead that they were just bones. That suggests there is hope. But someone had to speak life into them. Will that someone be you?

TAKE HEART

Do you speak life into others? Do you speak life into yourself?

TAKE ACTION

Words have power. Speak life to those around you.

Day 83

THE DANIEL FAST

Daniel then said to the guard..."Please test your servants for ten days: Give us nothing but vegetables to eat and water to drink. Then compare our appearance with that of the young men who eat the royal food, and treat your servants in accordance with what you see." So he agreed to this and tested them for ten days. At the end of the ten days they looked healthier and better nourished than any of the young men who ate the royal food.
—DANIEL 1:11–15

SOME PEOPLE GET really nervous when they hear the word *fasting*. Their stomachs start to growl, and they get visions of starving to death. This is not what fasting is about. You may have heard of the popular Daniel fast; perhaps you've even tried it. It is referencing a time in Daniel's life when he ate only water and vegetables and he thrived.

Now this is not a call for vegetarianism or veganism; it is a thought for you to consider. Would you drink water and eat only vegetables for ten days? Would you do it for the Lord as a form of worship and honor? Our responses to those questions are often very revealing.

TAKE HEART

What are you willing to give up for the Lord? Has food become an idol?

TAKE ACTION

Do a Daniel fast, consuming only water and vegetables for ten days. Journal and pray through this process.

Day 84
FACING THE FIERY FURNACE

So Shadrach, Meshach and Abednego came out of the fire,
and...the fire had not harmed their bodies, nor was a hair
of their heads singed; their robes were not scorched, and
there was no smell of fire on them. Then Nebuchadnezzar
said, "Praise be to the God of Shadrach, Meshach and
Abednego...! They trusted in him and defied the king's com-
mand and were willing to give up their lives rather than
serve or worship any god except their own God."
—DANIEL 3:26–28

THE BIBLE IS filled with amazing historical accounts of miraculous events. One of them is the story of Shadrach, Meshach,
and Abednego in Daniel 3. The king (authority) was mandating
they bow to a golden idol. The consequence if they didn't was
getting thrown into a fiery furnace. They took a public stand
for their beliefs, trusting that the Lord would rescue them. Yet
they also understood that they could die. Well, they survived
the fiery furnace without a scratch, and their boldness transformed the hearts of the king and countless others.

TAKE HEART

What do you think you would do if you faced the decision
Shadrach, Meshach, and Abednego encountered? What do
you do in less intense situations? Do you speak up?

TAKE ACTION

Find a way to be bold for Christ. Pray at lunch today; share a
scripture—just do one thing.

Day 85
NOT SO FAST

*I turned to the Lord God and pleaded with him in prayer
and petition, in fasting, and in sackcloth and ashes.*
—DANIEL 9:3

EARLIER WE TALKED about doing a Daniel fast, but there are lots of different ways to fast. One option to consider is called intermittent fasting, which helps us burn fat, lose weight, sleep better, think more clearly, and reduce inflammation, to name just a few benefits. This method is pretty straightforward: don't eat anything after 8 p.m., and eat your first meal of the next day at noon. This gives you sixteen hours of fasting. It is a great way to learn to turn to God instead of food.

TAKE HEART

Does intermittent fasting seem hard? Impossible? Scary? You can do it!

TAKE ACTION

Try intermittent fasting for one day. Be prepared and pre-*prayed*! It is a great way to see how food can be an idol in our lives.

Day 86
WAIT ON YOUR GOD

*But as for you, return to your God, hold fast to mercy
and justice, and wait on your God continually.*
—HOSEA 12:6, MEV

O H HOW WE don't like to wait on God. We want everything *now*. We want the quick fix. However, what often
appears as a "fix" is simply a covering over of the real issue.
If I have a fever (a God-given design to help me heal) and
take medicine to lower it, I have not fixed the problem.
Instead, in attempting to make myself more comfortable, I
have masked it.

We get annoyed when the internet is not fast, when home
delivery takes a few days, or when the line is long at the store.
It would do our hearts good to break free from the quick-
fix, "I want it now," and "what can I take to make myself feel
better" habits many of us have.

TAKE HEART

Jesus' timing is different than ours. I don't know why He created the timelines of healing He did; we can ask Him when
we get to heaven. Our job is not to figure it out so much as
to honor His wisdom. Where in your life do you try to rush
God?

TAKE ACTION

If you find yourself regularly frustrated with God and how
fast or slow He is doing what you want Him to do, it is probably time to reevaluate your position.

COME BACK TO GOD

Return, Israel, to the LORD your God. Your sins have been your downfall!...Who is wise? Let them realize these things. Who is discerning? Let them understand. The ways of the LORD are right; the righteous walk in them, but the rebellious stumble in them.
—HOSEA 14:1, 9

IT SEEMS LIKE our fallen human nature leads us astray endlessly. We talk ourselves into things, or we fall for cheap imitations. We think this world has what we desire and deserve, so we stumble time and time again. I once heard a person teach about smoking, and he mentioned that though people say it's hard to quit, it's actually harder to smoke because of the expense of buying cigarettes, the smell, the related health issues, and so on. He suggested that it's easier to just stop smoking!

It seems we often do this with God too. We want to see how much sin we can sneak into our lives (none). We see what we can get away with (but He knows all). And then we learn over and over that our best option is simply Him—to return to the Father.

TAKE HEART

Have you allowed or invited sloth, greed, or some other sin into your life?

TAKE ACTION

What do you need to just stop? Do it today.

Day 88

DREAM DREAMS

And afterward, I will pour out my Spirit on all people.
Your sons and daughters will prophesy, your old men
will dream dreams, your young men will see visions.
—JOEL 2:28

DO YOU STILL have dreams? Do you still believe that God is on the move? Do you still have a zeal and expectancy for what the Lord is doing? Some amazing attributes of God are His steadfastness and relentlessness. He never stops. He's always at work; nothing gets by Him. He never takes a vacation, He never sleeps, and we never have to worry about Him dropping the ball. But we do. We get comfortable. We get satisfied. We get stuck in ruts. We get scared. We get old.

The Lord is an endless Creator, and He is still creating in you—every second! He just created another beat in your heart, another thought in your mind. Expect the Lord to do a new thing in you today!

TAKE HEART

Do you still desire and expect new and fresh experiences with the Lord?

TAKE ACTION

Mix it up. Read a new book or listen to new sermon. Challenge yourself to step out of your comfort zone. Try praying out loud or getting on your knees. Shake yourself out of routine. Sometimes we get in a rut.

Day 89
GIVER OF LIFE

This is what the LORD says...: "Seek me and live;
do not seek Bethel, do not go to Gilgal, do not
journey to Beersheba. For Gilgal will surely go into
exile, and Bethel will be reduced to nothing.
—AMOS 5:4–5

GOD IS THE only one who gives life. In all of time, with all our money, scientific advancements, and research, humans have never made a single cell. We can clone and manipulate cells, but we cannot create life. Only God can. So if you want life—real life—there is only one place to go and only one person to seek: the Creator of it all, including your life.

Seek Him. Nothing else brings life, especially not our own ambitions. The Bible says, "There is a way that appears to be right, but in the end it leads to death" (Prov. 14:12). Choose life, not death.

TAKE HEART

Is God alone enough for you? Or do you just want things from Him as though He's an Amazon delivery, a genie in a bottle, or Santa Claus?

TAKE ACTION

Take the next few minutes to go outside or to a window and just look at what God created. Then look in a mirror. Let those be reminders that He's worth seeking!

Day 90
URGENCY

The day of the LORD is near for all nations. As you have done, it will be done to you; your deeds will return upon your own head.
—OBADIAH 15

TOMORROW IS NOT guaranteed. As a matter of fact, not even the next second is promised. We will reap what we sow. Our actions, thoughts, and choices have implications and consequences—both good and bad.

There are countless sermons about "If you died today, do you know where you're going?" Now I believe this is a critical question. But if you *don't* die today or tomorrow, are you living a life worthy of what Jesus died for? Are you representing Christ well as a parent, spouse, friend, boss, neighbor, etc.? Don't wait!

TAKE HEART

What is an area where you are not as Christlike as you should be?

TAKE ACTION

What is one thing that you can do today to represent Jesus well: offer an apology, forgive someone, be generous? Do it.

YOU CAN RUN, BUT YOU CAN'T HIDE

But Jonah ran away from the LORD and headed for Tarshish. He went down to Joppa, where he found a ship bound for that port. After paying the fare, he went aboard and sailed for Tarshish to flee from the LORD.
—JONAH 1:3

GOD HAS PLANS for you. Notice I said *God* has plans. Some of us run from those plans, and we suffer accordingly. Sometimes the plans God has for us are not the ones we want. But they are His plans. Jonah did not like the people God asked him to serve and share the truth with. Jonah didn't think they deserved it. But God did.

God created you for a reason. Your life matters. You can never outrun God. Surrender your plans to His.

TAKE HEART

Have you ever run from God? Are you still running in any particular area? Why?

TAKE ACTION

Have you ever resisted something God asked you to do? It's not too late. Do something to change that today. Whether it's helping a homeless person, engaging in a random act of kindness, or praying for a coworker or a family member, do whatever the Lord is encouraging you to do.

TELL ME WHAT I WANT TO HEAR

*If a liar and deceiver comes and says, "I will
prophesy for you plenty of wine and beer," that
would be just the prophet for this people!*
—MICAH 2:11

FALSE PROPHETS ARE still out there, and they speak in a variety of ways and on a plethora of topics. They can be posting on social media or standing in a pulpit speaking about fad diets, bio hacks, magic cures, and the like. We are often attracted to or fall for these claims because we want more by doing less. Be careful whom you listen to, and check their words and actions against Scripture. As the old saying goes, "If it's too good to be true, it probably is."

TAKE HEART

Do you guard your mind and heart against worldly or fleshly things? Do you like your ears to be tickled to justify certain sinful practices?

TAKE ACTION

We are to test all things against God's Word. Review some of the habits or teachings you have been consuming. Are they aligned with the Word of God, or do they seem to be more aligned with the world?

Day 93
A GOD LIKE YOU

Who is a God like you, who pardons sin and forgives the transgression of the remnant of his inheritance? You do not stay angry forever but delight to show mercy. You will again have compassion on us; you will tread our sins underfoot and hurl all our iniquities into the depths of the sea.
—MICAH 7:18–19

IT IS ALMOST impossible for us to fathom how God forgives and loves us. Our human minds and hearts that take offense, hold grudges, and judge others simply cannot imagine the love of God for us.

God is not like us. It is critical that we remind ourselves of this daily, receive His grace and mercy, and live in thanksgiving and worship of such a marvelous King.

TAKE HEART

What overwhelms you about God's love?

TAKE ACTION

Review some of your relationships and how you are toward others. Are you easily offended? Are you slow to forgive? Does anyone come to mind you need to reach out to? Do it today.

THE LORD IS GOOD, JUST, AND FAIR

The LORD is a jealous and avenging God; the LORD takes ven-
geance...on his foes and vents his wrath against his ene-
mies. The LORD is slow to anger but great in power; the LORD
will not leave the guilty unpunished....The LORD is good, a
refuge in times of trouble. He cares for those who trust in
him but...he will pursue his foes into the realm of darkness.
—NAHUM 1:2–3, 7–8

WE LOVE TO hear, read, and sing about the goodness of God. And there is so much goodness to talk about! However, we need to keep other aspects of His love and goodness close to our hearts and minds. God is never OK with sin. His grace and mercy never endorse sinful lives—ever. The wages of sin are death. Both the Old and New Testaments give many examples of the wrath of God. Here is the question for us: Is there known sin in our lives that we have become OK with, that we have stopped contending against? Just because we're OK with it doesn't mean God is.

TAKE HEART

God is relentless. He wants your whole heart. He loves you too much to leave you in your sin. Is there an area you are struggling with? Name it.

TAKE ACTION

Now, take that issue to the Lord in prayer. Earnestly seek His help. Consider including trusted friends to help you and provide accountability. It matters that you take sin seriously.

Day 95

HOW LONG, LORD, MUST
I CALL FOR HELP?

How long, LORD, must I call for help, but you do not listen?
—HABAKKUK 1:2

W E KNOW GOD is a good God. We know He hears our prayers. We know He is fair and just, but we sure don't like His schedule sometimes—or even most of the time. Habakkuk expressed his frustrations boldly. And God answered clearly. At the conclusion of this book is a frustrated prophet who sees God more clearly and surrenders to His ways.

You may have made some positive changes. You may be getting closer to God, yet it may seem like evil is winning. Many people think good guys finish last. But God reminds us that His perspective is different and infinitely bigger than ours.

TAKE HEART

Do you have frustrations or doubts? Have you taken them to God?

TAKE ACTION

Habakkuk 2:2–3 says, "Then the LORD replied: 'Write down the revelation and make it plain on tablets so that a herald may run with it. For the revelation awaits an appointed time; it speaks of the end and will not prove false. Though it linger, wait for it; it will certainly come and will not delay.'" Notice He says to write the revelation. Do you journal? It's a great habit. Start today. Write down your thoughts and questions to God, as well as His responses.

HE IS MIGHTY TO SAVE

*Fear not, O Zion; let not your hands be slack. The LORD
your God is in your midst, a Mighty One, who will save.
He will rejoice over you with gladness, He will renew you
with His love, He will rejoice over you with singing.*
—ZEPHANIAH 3:16–17, MEV

THERE IS A tension when we're walking out our lives as believers. We're surrendering our lives to an almighty God. We know that sin leads to death, that we are called to live righteous and godly lives, that we are called to die to self, pick up our cross, etc. And we know that God is mighty to save, He takes delight in us, and He will guard us with His love. However, these promises are to those He has chosen, those who seek His face. In today's culture, even inside the church, we are often so focused on ourselves that we lose the perspective of worshipping the mighty God. We desperately need to fear God. Fear of God is the beginning of wisdom.

TAKE HEART

Do you fear God?

TAKE ACTION

Reflect on your foundational view of God. How would you describe it? It is critical because it leads to your actions. For instance, I will know how much you believe in prayer when you tell me how much you pray.

Day 97
GOD FIRST

Now this is what the LORD Almighty says: "Give careful thought to your ways. You have planted much, but harvested little. You eat, but never have enough. You drink, but never have your fill. You put on clothes, but are not warm. You earn wages, only to put them in a purse with holes in it."
—HAGGAI 1:5–6

WE HEAR A lot nowadays about self-care, "me time," loving ourselves, etc. Although these may have some temporary value and some "feel-good" moments, it is easy to forget God and others and be too self-focused. God reminds us that we must serve Him first. This perspective is seldom even discussed in church today. We may give lip service to serving God, but often our lives are mostly about us—the opposite of what God has called us to do. We want a little more. We shy away from asking ourselves how we can serve others. When it comes to caring for ourselves, do we too often see self-care as a form of worship to God or stewardship rather than an issue of pride, vanity, or selfishness?

TAKE HEART

Why do you take care of yourself—mind, body, and spirit? Is your answer aligned with Scripture?

TAKE ACTION

The next time you're exercising, taking a Sabbath, or eating, intentionally surrender to God. Give Him the glory.

Day 98
THE FUTURE

The LORD will be king over the whole earth. On that day
there will be one LORD, and his name the only name.
—ZECHARIAH 14:9

SCRIPTURE INCLUDES MANY references to God's omniscience—His all-knowing abilities—and several prophets and prophesies give us a glimpse into what lies ahead. However, no one really knows when Christ will return, and none of us know when our last breaths will be. We all know people who have died suddenly as a result of either accidents or health tragedies. Only God knows the lengths of our days. Yet we often live one of two ways: reckless and self-centered, with little regard for the bodies God gave us, or in such fear of dying that we create an idol of healthy living. Both miss the mark. We are to live fearless lives for Christ, serving Him through our minds, bodies, and spirits.

TAKE HEART

Have you missed the mark? Are you living a selfish, fearful life?

TAKE ACTION

Reflect on the priorities in your daily schedule. Do an audit of your time. Does your reality reflect a person who loves and serves God first?

ARE YOU ROBBING GOD?

"I the LORD do not change....Ever since the time of your ances-
tors you have turned away from my decrees and have
not kept them. Return to me, and I will return to you," says
the LORD Almighty. But you ask, "How are we to return?"
Will a mere mortal rob God? Yet you rob Me. But you
ask, "How are we robbing you?" In tithes and offerings.
—MALACHI 3:6–8, MEV

SOMETIMES WE GET uncomfortable discussing tithes and offerings. What I want to offer here is this: We are called to offer up our lives and bodies as offerings. Our lives are not our own. They were bought for a price. Jesus went to the cross for you. He took your place. His life was a ransom. This was a dramatic and incredible act that changed the world. Let us understand the weight of this action and live accordingly.

TAKE HEART

When you think about Christ taking your place on the cross and about offering your life to Him, how does it make you feel?

TAKE ACTION

Do you tithe? What do you sacrifice for the Lord?

THE FAITHFUL FEW—THE REMNANT

*Then those who feared the LORD talked with each other,
and the LORD listened and heard. A scroll of remembrance was written in his presence concerning those
who feared the LORD and honored his name.*
—MALACHI 3:16

A LL GOD'S PROMISES are true. However, the nature of your relationship with the Lord will determine what you experience. There are people who will receive God's blessing and favor and those who will receive His wrath. Which one are you? Do you fear the Lord and honor His name? Is He your focus, your guiding light, the lens you navigate the world through? Are you a "Jesus freak," or do you blend in too well?

I once heard of a believer who was not living for Christ. When he finally decided to serve God completely and put God first in his life, he told his neighbors about it. They were all shocked. They had had no idea he was a Christian.

TAKE HEART

Would your neighbors—or even your friends—be surprised to learn you love Jesus?

TAKE ACTION

Heed Christ's warning to fear the Lord (Prov. 9:10). You want to be a part of the remnant! You want to make the cut. Surrender everything to Jesus; it's all His anyway.

Day 101

WITH CHILD FROM THE HOLY SPIRIT

This is how the birth of Jesus the Messiah came about: His mother Mary was pledged to be married to Joseph, but before they came together, she was found to be pregnant through the Holy Spirit.
—MATTHEW 1:18

THE FIRST "MEDICAL miracle" we read about in the New Testament is the virgin Mary becoming pregnant supernaturally. This miracle had never happened before and hasn't happened since. It's a miracle that defies all medical, natural, and physiological laws. It defied the moral code and caused a whole lot of problems. It's the miracle of all miracles. The Holy Spirit did the impossible!

And He still does. As we begin our journey into the New Testament, I want to challenge your faith in this area. God can do and still does miracles—specifically and purposefully. And you are included in that. Do you need a miracle? I know just the guy. And He came to this world in a very miraculous way! (It was even a home birth, with no doctors, drugs, or vaccines.)

TAKE HEART

Do you believe in miracles? Do you believe God would do one for you? Why or why not?

TAKE ACTION

Have you ever experienced a miracle? Take a moment to relive that story. What is one miracle you need now? Ask God for it!

Day 102

BAPTISM BY FIRE

I baptize you with water for repentance. But after me comes one
who is more powerful than I, whose sandals I am not worthy
to carry. He will baptize you with the Holy Spirit and fire.
—MATTHEW 3:11

YOU MAY HAVE been baptized in water as an infant or as an adult. However, maybe you have not been baptized with the Holy Spirit, which ignites His fire inside you. If this describes you, or you're not sure, I urge you to go after this with the Lord. Baptism with the Holy Spirit and His fire changes everything! If you are feeling stuck, scared, bored, or dead, you need to be baptized in the Spirit. It's *the* game changer. Pray to the Lord about this baptism. Find a church that baptizes in the Holy Spirit. It may seem weird or crazy to you, but Jesus doesn't fit in a box. Remember, He's a God of miracles. He came into the world like no one else, and He can do whatever, whenever, and however He sees fit.

TAKE HEART

How do you feel about the baptism of the Holy Spirit and His fire?

TAKE ACTION

If you have not been baptized in the Holy Spirit, I can't encourage you enough to do so.

DESIGNED TO HEAL

Day 103
TEMPTATION

Then Jesus was led by the Spirit into the wilderness to be tempted by the devil. After fasting forty days and forty nights, he was hungry.
—MATTHEW 4:1–2

THIS IS SO critical. Immediately after Jesus was baptized and the heavens literally opened, He was *led by the Spirit* to be tempted by the devil! Did you read that? He was baptized by the Holy Spirit, and immediately that same Holy Spirit led Him to the desert for forty days of fasting and temptation. Surrendering your life—everything—to Jesus is often a wild adventure. God is the ultimate creator; He gives you every breath, every heartbeat. Following Jesus can take you to the desert, face to face with the devil, but here is the good news: you would never be able to handle the devil without Jesus! The enemy has been defeated. No matter what you're facing, through Christ all things are possible.

TAKE HEART

Have you been tempted by the devil? Do you get frustrated in the desert? Or do you know you have the Lord with you?

TAKE ACTION

Temptation is not an excuse for sinning or living an ungodly lifestyle. It's a reason to cling to Jesus. Don't go in unprepared. Honor the Holy Spirit.

Day 104
JESUS HEALS THE SICK

Jesus went throughout Galilee, teaching in their syna-
gogues, proclaiming the good news of the kingdom, and
healing every disease and sickness among the people.
News about him spread all over Syria, and people brought
to him all who were ill with various diseases, those suf-
fering severe pain, the demon-possessed, those having
seizures, and the paralyzed; and he healed them.
—MATTHEW 4:23–24

WHEN JESUS STARTED His earthly ministry, He went out
teaching with the first disciples, and the Bible says they
were healing *all* diseases. All means all! Total. Every condition you can think of—physical and otherwise—was healed.

Has culture affected your faith in what God will heal? Is
stage IV cancer too much for Him? Schizophrenia? Seizures?
Birth defects? Depression? Infertility? Why? You may need
to read this passage daily for several months. Meditate on it
every day. He can and does heal all diseases and afflictions.

TAKE HEART

Do you believe God can heal you? Today? Now? What action
does your belief cause you to take?

TAKE ACTION

Read today's passage ten times a day for ten days. Be on the
lookout for healing miracles.

Day 105

LET YOUR LIGHT SHINE!

*Let your light shine before others, that they may see
your good deeds and glorify your Father in heaven.*
—MATTHEW 5:16

RESEARCH HAS SHOWN that our bodies glow and radiate light that our human eyes cannot see.[1] We are called to shine—literally. The question is, How bright are you shining? We are commanded in Matthew 5 to be the light of the world, let our light be seen, and not hide it under a bowl. We do not need to hide our faith or play small; we are called to be bold and courageous.

(Side note: Have you ever heard someone tell a pregnant woman that she is "glowing"? I wonder if this is because she is literally carrying a miracle inside her.)

TAKE HEART

Are you glowing? Are you shining? Why or why not?

TAKE ACTION

When is the last time you shared your faith? I have heard that 95 percent of Christians have never led another person to Christ. This is a sad statistic. We know Jesus is the one who saves, but He uses people to share the good news. Share your faith with someone today.

ANGER

Anyone who is angry with a brother or sister will be subject to judgment. Again, anyone who says to a brother or sister, "Raca," is answerable to the court. And anyone who says, "You fool!" will be in danger of the fire of hell. Therefore, if you are offering your gift at the altar and there remember that your brother or sister has something against you...first go and be reconciled to them; then come and offer your gift.
—MATTHEW 5:22–24

WHEN IT COMES to health, wellness, and healing, we typically focus on foods, exercise, detox, and treatments. We don't often discuss the role of emotions such as fear, anger, and unforgiveness. Yet these emotions can be as dangerous as other lifestyle areas, and the Lord is very clear about this.

Do you struggle with anger? Have you engaged with the Lord and Scripture to take practical steps to change? Anger can mess you up worse than cigarettes. But Jesus can help you.

TAKE HEART

Do you struggle with any areas emotionally? Are you quick to become angry or harbor unforgiveness? Are you impatient, rude, crude, lazy, or unkind? God desires to set you free!

TAKE ACTION

Pick the one area you struggle with the most, and take it to the Lord. Listen to some sermons, or talk with some wise elders about tools and scriptures to help you break free from these emotional strongholds and bear the fruit of the Spirit.

FASTING

*When you fast, do not look somber as the hypocrites do, for
they disfigure their faces to show others they are fasting.
Truly I tell you, they have received their reward in full. But
when you fast, put oil on your head and wash your face.*
—MATTHEW 6:16–17

WE HEAR A lot about fasting, and much of it is great. There
are many ways to fast and some wonderful books about
fasting. But here is what I want to explore: Don't tell anyone
about your fasting. Don't post it on social media. Don't complain about it. Don't brag about it. Don't whine about it. Just
fast. It is between you and the Lord—period.

As wellness has become more popular, there is a tendency
for pride, vanity, and self-righteousness to surface. Make
a promise to God and yourself to not post, brag, or complain about your worship and stewardship to the Lord. No
one except the Lord needs to see your workout picture and
smoothie selfie.

TAKE HEART

Does what I said in today's devotional convict or offend you?
Why?

TAKE ACTION

No more posting or telling others about your health and
wellness. Celebrate other victories. Share edifying content.
Remember, life is not all about you.

TREASURES IN HEAVEN

*Do not store up for yourselves treasures on earth....But
store up for yourselves treasures in heaven....For where
your treasure is, there your heart will be also....No one can
serve two masters. Either you will hate the one and love
the other, or you will be devoted to the one and despise
the other. You cannot serve both God and money.*
—MATTHEW 6:19–21, 24

HERE WE GO. This one might sting. The Lord is very clear
that we cannot serve two masters. Many of us are chasing
the world. We are building our little empires of "just a little
more." A lifestyle of burning the candle at both ends as we try
to keep up with the Joneses will eventually destroy us. The Lord
says it's not worth it. Solomon, known for his wisdom, warned
us against this as well. Materialism and the American dream
have perverted many of our hearts. Seek God for sanctification
and more of Him.

TAKE HEART

Are you spending more time storing treasures in heaven or on
earth? What do you think Jesus would say about your priorities? What can you remove? What needs to go?

TAKE ACTION

Pick one thing to prune. Make it sting a bit; that's a good sign
it's taking up too much space. Ask the Lord what you should
do. It's time to do some housecleaning in your life. You cannot
serve two masters.

Day 109

OPEN THE EYES

*The light of the body is the eye. Therefore, if your eye
is clear, your whole body will be full of light.*
—MATTHEW 6:22, MEV

THE HUMAN EYE'S resolution is about the equivalent of
576 megapixels.[1] Leave it to God—the human eye that
we often take for granted blows any current camera or technology away in terms of megapixels. And remember, your
eyes formed as you were being knit together in your mother's
womb (Ps. 139:13). No drug, pill, or doctor was involved in
creating this magnificent organ—just God. Incredible!

TAKE HEART

We tend to focus on the problems instead of the miracles.
The fact that we can see at all is amazing. The fact that we
have eyes that can see better than any man-made camera is
incredible.

TAKE ACTION

If you had a $10,000 camera or a $500,000 car, you would
probably take good care of it. Yet we have these priceless
bodies, and we often treat them like they are disposable cam-
eras. See your body as a priceless gift from God.

Day 110
DO NOT BE ANXIOUS

*Do not worry, saying, "What shall we eat?" or '"What
shall we drink?" or "What shall we wear?" For the pagans
run after all these things, and your heavenly Father knows
that you need them. But seek first his kingdom and his righteousness, and all these things will be given to you as well.
Therefore do not worry about tomorrow, for tomorrow will
worry about itself. Each day has enough trouble of its own.*
—Matthew 6:31–34

WHAT A CHALLENGING passage of Scripture that speaks
right to today's times. Several studies have revealed
what an anxious, stressed, fearful people we have become.
The Lord reminds us how much He loves us and implores
us to look around and not fear or worry. He even says that
we should not worry about dying. Amazing. So what do we
do? He tells us: seek first His kingdom, and all else will be
added. Our role is simple: *seek God*. He decides what our indi-
vidual portions will be. There is such profound and powerful
wisdom in this passage.

TAKE HEART

Are you anxious? Do you worry? If so, what do you worry
about? What does the Bible say about that issue?

TAKE ACTION

List all your fears, anxieties, and worries. Be honest. Just
list them. Now, read and reread exactly what Jesus said in
Matthew 6:28–34. Pray, repent, and seek His kingdom!

THE INCURABLE DISEASE
OF LEPROSY—GONE

A man with leprosy came and knelt before him and said, "Lord, if you are willing, you can make me clean." Jesus reached out his hand and touched the man. "I am willing," he said. "Be clean!" Immediately he was cleansed of his leprosy.
—MATTHEW 8:2–3

WE DON'T HEAR a lot about leprosy these days, but I have actually been to a leper colony in Africa. It was a small hut in the middle of the desert, where men, women, and children were sent if they had the contagious disease. Back in the day, leprosy was essentially a death sentence physically and even culturally because you were considered unclean. Your life was over. But Jesus, fearless Jesus. The man with leprosy approached the Lord and asked Him for healing. Don't miss this point: the leprous man took action. He believed the Lord could heal him. So he went to Jesus and asked the Lord without a big show or fanfare. Jesus responded by simply taking his hand and saying, "Be clean," and the man was healed instantly.

Jesus touches the untouchable. He heals the sick. He hears our prayers.

TAKE HEART

Do you boldly approach the Lord? Do you believe He can heal you?

TAKE ACTION

Pray for someone, expecting God to hear and answer.

YOU ARE A CANCER KILLER!

Jesus reached out his hand and touched the man. "I am willing,"
he said. "Be clean!" Immediately he was cleansed of his leprosy.
—MATTHEW 8:3

CANCER. THE WORD alone causes fear for many. But here is some good news: God has provided amazing immune systems that are constantly finding and destroying cells in our bodies that could develop into cancers. This is great news! Yes, *your immune system killed cancer today*! God has designed our bodies to daily kill thousands of cells that potentially carry what so many fear.

The Bible does not specifically name cancer, but it gives numerous examples of incurable diseases being healed! Take comfort in that fact.

TAKE HEART

Are your lifestyle choices helping your body kill cancer?

TAKE ACTION

Give thanks to God for the natural, innate immune system He gave you!

HEALED BY THE FAITH
OF SOMEONE ELSE

*A centurion came to him, asking for help. "Lord," he said, "my
servant lies at home paralyzed, suffering terribly." Jesus said to
him, "Shall I come and heal him?" The centurion replied, "Lord,
I do not deserve to have you come under my roof. But just say
the word, and my servant will be healed...." When Jesus heard
this, he was amazed and said to those following him, "Truly I tell
you, I have not found anyone in Israel with such great faith."...
Then Jesus said to the centurion, "Go! Let it be done just as you
believed it would." And his servant was healed at that moment.*
—MATTHEW 8:5–8, 10, 13

THIS IS ANOTHER amazing story of healing through Jesus.
Remember, Jesus heals more than just physical bodies; we
are to bring *all* things to Him in prayer. But I love this story
because it was the *centurion's* faith that led to the healing.
Imagine that your friend is at home paralyzed. You go to Jesus
on his behalf and ask for healing, and the next thing you know,
your friend at home is walking around! This is exactly what
happened. Jesus said, "Let it be done," and the man was healed!

TAKE HEART

Do you pray for others' healing? Do you have faith that would
move Jesus?

TAKE ACTION

Get on your knees (literally), and pray for some of your sick
friends (or enemies).

Day 114

JESUS HEALS EVEN IN-LAWS

When Jesus came into Peter's house, he saw Peter's mother-in-law lying in bed with a fever. He touched her hand and the fever left her, and she got up and began to wait on him. When evening came, many who were demon-possessed were brought to him, and he drove out the spirits with a word and healed all the sick. This was to fulfill what was spoken through the prophet Isaiah: "He took up our infirmities and bore our diseases."
—MATTHEW 8:14–17

SOMETIMES THE BIBLE just makes you laugh. Peter's mother-in-law was sick with a fever. Jesus healed her, and she hopped up and began to work. If Jesus can heal even mothers-in-law, then there's nothing He can't do! Just kidding. But I love that Jesus healed something as simple as a fever.

Later that night people came with many different issues, and all were healed. Let me ask you this: When you have a fever, whom or what do you trust more—God or painkillers? Some of us have replaced our faith in God with faith in pills.

TAKE HEART

Do you have lots of medications? Why? Do you take steps to give your body what it needs to heal? Have you talked with health-care practitioners who may have opinions that are different from what has become standard medical practice?

TAKE ACTION

After reviewing all the medications you use, talk to God about them and see what He has to say.

Day 115
JESUS CALMS THE STORM

A furious storm came up on the lake, so that the waves swept over the boat. But Jesus was sleeping. The disciples went and woke him, saying, "Lord, save us! We're going to drown!" He replied, "You of little faith, why are you so afraid?" Then he got up and rebuked the winds and the waves, and it was completely calm. The men were amazed and asked, "What kind of man is this? Even the winds and the waves obey him!"
—MATTHEW 8:24–27

SOMETIMES YOU HAVE to slow down when you read the Bible and put yourself in the moment. Imagine this: You are a seasoned fisherman. You're out in a boat, and there's a horrible storm—so bad you think you're going to die. Jesus is on the boat *sleeping*. You're scared and mad. So you wake up the miracle worker, who says, "Come on, why are you scared? You have such little faith." Then He speaks to the storm, and it's over. The disciples' minds were blown, and if you're like me, yours would be too.

You may be in a terrible storm, but Jesus is right there with you. He's not worried at all. Neither should you be.

TAKE HEART

Jesus can do miracles in any domain. Do you believe that? Do you wake Jesus up to help you?

TAKE ACTION

What impossible issues do you need to pray about? Write them down, and pray daily until you see results.

NOT EVERYONE WILL BE HAPPY ABOUT YOUR HEALING

When he arrived...in the region of the Gadarenes, two demon-possessed men coming from the tombs met him...."What do you want with us, Son of God?" they shouted....The demons begged Jesus, "If you drive us out, send us into the herd of pigs." He said to them, "Go!" So they came out and went into the pigs, and the whole herd rushed down the steep bank into the lake and died in the water. Those tending the pigs ran off...and reported all this....Then the whole town went out to meet Jesus...[and] pleaded with him to leave their region.
—MATTHEW 8:28–29, 31–34

WE COULD DISCUSS so much about this story. But here is one point to ponder: this miracle inconvenienced others and upset them so much they chased Jesus out of town. When you choose a healthy lifestyle and reach your ideal weight, gain energy, and no longer take prescription medication every day, not everyone will be happy for you. But if you trust God with your health and give your body what it needs, you can expect miraculous results.

TAKE HEART

If Jesus performed a miracle for someone you don't like, how would you respond?

TAKE ACTION

Do you believe God can heal your body as you make healthy choices? I challenge you to surrender your health to Him.

RISE

*Some men brought to him a paralyzed man, lying on a
mat. When Jesus saw their faith, he said to the man, "Take
heart, son; your sins are forgiven." At this, some of the
teachers of the law said to themselves, "This fellow is blaspheming!" Knowing their thoughts, Jesus said, "...Which is
easier: to say, 'Your sins are forgiven,' or to say, 'Get up and
walk'?..." So he said to the paralyzed man, "Get up, take your
mat and go home." Then the man got up and went home.*
—Matthew 9:2–7

THIS AMAZING MIRACLE has a deep lesson for us. Here is
the scene: Jesus meets some guys carrying their paralyzed
friend to Him to be healed. Seeing their faith, Jesus says, "Son,
your sins are forgiven." This angered some people who didn't
think Jesus was divine and had the authority to forgive sins. The
next part is a mic drop. Jesus asks them, "What is harder: to forgive his sin or have him rise and walk?" Then He heals the man.

You may find it easier to believe Jesus can forgive your sins
and give you eternal life than to heal you physically. But the
truth is, He has the power to do both!

TAKE HEART

Why do many people easily accept that Jesus forgives their
sins but struggle to believe He will heal them?

TAKE ACTION

Ponder how amazing the forgiveness of sins is and what that
affords you.

IT IS *NEVER* TOO LATE

*When Jesus entered the synagogue leader's house and
saw the noisy crowd and people playing pipes, he
said, "Go away. The girl is not dead but asleep." But they
laughed at him. After the crowd had been put outside, he
went in and took the girl by the hand, and she got up.*
—MATTHEW 9:23–25

I ENCOURAGE YOU TO read all of Matthew 9:18–26 because it
is an amazing story. A little girl died. The dad found Jesus,
believing He could heal his daughter. But what we didn't read
in today's passage is that when Jesus was on the way to resurrect this child, a woman who had struggled for twelve years
with a bleeding problem delayed Him. She believed if she
could simply touch Him, she would be healed. So she fought
her way through the crowd and touched Him, and Jesus said
her faith had made her well. He then arrived at the dead
child's home, and everyone said it was too late. But Jesus took
the girl's hand and brought her back to life. Glory to God for
the faith these people displayed!

TAKE HEART

Have you given up? Do you think it's too late? If you'd been
suffering for twelve years, would you still be chasing Jesus? If
your child was dead, would you think it was too late?

TAKE ACTION

Pray for someone or yourself about a long-standing problem.
Resurrect some dreams you gave up on!

Day 119
I WAS BLIND, BUT NOW I SEE

*As Jesus went on from there, two blind men followed him,
calling out, "Have mercy on us, Son of David!" When he had
gone indoors, the blind men came to him, and he asked them,
"Do you believe that I am able to do this?" "Yes, Lord," they
replied. Then he touched their eyes and said, "According to
your faith let it be done to you"; and their sight was restored.*
—MATTHEW 9:27–30

HERE IS ANOTHER incredible miracle with something to
teach us. Two blind guys hear about Jesus. They desire
to be healed, and they believe Jesus can do it. They seek Him.
They beg Jesus to have mercy on them and heal them. He asks
whether they believe He can heal them. They say, "Yes, Lord."
He touches their eyes, and they are healed.

What an intense encounter. I love the conversation Jesus
had with these men who desired healing. Their faith led them
to take action, and Jesus responded by doing the miraculous.

TAKE HEART

Are you chasing after Jesus, begging Him to have mercy on
you? Why or why not? What does that reveal about your faith?

TAKE ACTION

If you are a believer, the Holy Spirit resides in you. You have
direct access *right now* to the King of kings! Seek Him now!

DEALING WITH DEMONS

*A man who was demon-possessed and could not talk was
brought to Jesus. And when the demon was driven out, the man
who had been mute spoke. The crowd was amazed and said,
"Nothing like this has ever been seen in Israel." But the Pharisees
said, "It is by the prince of demons that he drives out demons."*
—MATTHEW 9:32–34

FOR SOME PEOPLE, talking about demons, deliverance,
and casting out spirits is uncomfortable or taboo. Why?
In the Scriptures, it is incredibly common to read stories
about demons and their influence on people. It's throughout
the Bible, from the very beginning to the end. We would be
remiss to not acknowledge there is evil, there is a devil, and
there are powers and principalities we must be prepared to
deal with. The only way to deal with them is through Jesus.

In today's passage, Jesus cast out a demon from a man who
was so tormented he could not even speak. Jesus commanded
the demon to leave, and a man was set free. Victory!

TAKE HEART

Do you believe people still need help being set free from spiritual strongholds?

TAKE ACTION

It's possible you have not addressed the demonic aspect of certain issues; even some health issues can have spiritual roots.
Reflect on some areas you are struggling with, and ask the Lord
to reveal whether you are dealing with a demonic stronghold.

Day 121

HE HAD COMPASSION ON THEM

*Jesus went through all the towns and villages, teaching
in their synagogues, proclaiming the good news of the
kingdom and healing every disease and sickness. When
he saw the crowds, he had compassion on them, because
they were harassed and helpless, like sheep without a shepherd. Then he said to his disciples, "The harvest is plentiful but the workers are few. Ask the Lord of the harvest,
therefore, to send out workers into his harvest field."*
—MATTHEW 9:35–38

THIS IS AN incredible scene. As healing miracles happened
and the crowd grew, Jesus saw all these hurting, suffering
lost sheep and had compassion. The passage says He healed
every disease and affliction! And Jesus said, "The harvest is
plentiful but the workers are few."

Although it's impossible to fully understand how Jesus
sees things, I imagine Him looking out over the thousands of
scared, hurting, lost people and desperately wanting them to
understand how great God is, how big and mighty. I believe
Jesus was saying to them—and to us today—that if they could
grasp this, they could not only be healed but also help serve
others in His name. Be Christlike, Christian.

TAKE HEART

Are you a laborer? Or do you just want Jesus to do it all?

TAKE ACTION

Serve others. Be the hands and feet of Jesus to someone!

HE KNOWS THE HAIRS
ON YOUR HEAD!

Even the very hairs of your head are all numbered.
—MATTHEW 10:30

INVENTOR THOMAS EDISON once said, "The doctor of the future will give no medicine but will interest his patient in the care of the human frame, in diet and in the cause and prevention of disease."[1] I have always loved this quote. Imagine if health care were actually practiced this way.

The good news is, you can decide to operate in this model today. Many people live lifestyles that do not require drugs; rather, they focus on caring for the bodies God gave them. Remember, this is the same God who *created* you!

TAKE HEART

Do you think it's possible to avoid diseases and prescriptions just by caring for our bodies? Do you think health care would be better off if we focused on the quote above?

TAKE ACTION

Review the model of health care you are participating in. Does it align with your values and beliefs? If not, find one that does.

HEALING ON THE SABBATH

*A man with a shriveled hand was [at the synagogue].
Looking for a reason to bring charges against Jesus, they
asked him, "Is it lawful to heal on the Sabbath?" He said to
them, "If any of you has a sheep and it falls into a pit on the
Sabbath, will you not...lift it out? How much more valuable
is a person than a sheep! Therefore it is lawful to do good
on the Sabbath." Then he said to the man, "Stretch out your
hand." So he stretched it out and it was completely restored.*
—MATTHEW 12:9–13

JESUS HATES RELIGION. He is about relationship. Jesus also
does not follow a formula. This drove the Pharisees crazy,
and if we are honest, it can bother us too. Honoring the Sabbath is a critical aspect of the Christian walk. However, when
a man in need approached Jesus, He healed him even though
it was the Sabbath. Here's a thought: Maybe one reason Jesus
healed the man is that, to Him, healing isn't work. It's as natural as breathing for Him. He does it all the time.

TAKE HEART

Do you ever think, "This is too much to ask or to pray for"?

TAKE ACTION

Put people over rules. Don't be so rigid. Volunteer. Or consider stopping and praying with a homeless person. Find a
way to serve others.

HE GAVE THANKS AND THEN FED ALL FIVE THOUSAND!

Taking the five loaves and the two fish and looking up to heaven, he gave thanks and broke the loaves. Then he gave them to the disciples, and the disciples gave them to the people. They all ate and were satisfied, and the disciples picked up twelve basketfuls of broken pieces that were left over. The number of those who ate was about five thousand men, besides women and children.
—MATTHEW 14:19–21

IMAGINE THAT YOU just found out your friend was murdered and that you have thousands of people following you who all want something from you. Sounds like a stressful day, right? This is what Jesus was facing. John the Baptist had just been killed, yet Jesus didn't put His pain over others' needs. He continued to minister. First He healed the sick. Then He fed over five thousand people with five loaves of bread and two fish.

Jesus is never too busy, too tired, or too depleted of resources to meet our needs. Remember, He's the God who made everything from nothing. Meeting our needs is not hard for Him. But notice what He did before He fed everyone: He lifted what He had to heaven and gave thanks.

TAKE HEART

Do you give thanks to God for what you have?

TAKE ACTION

Write a list of fifty things you are thankful for, and then thank God for them. Then write fifty more.

WATER WALKER

Shortly before dawn Jesus went out to them, walking on the lake. When the disciples saw him walking on the lake, they were terrified....But Jesus immediately said to them: "Take courage! It is I. Don't be afraid." "Lord, if it's you," Peter replied, "tell me to come to you on the water." "Come," he said. Then Peter got down out of the boat, walked on the water and came toward Jesus. But when he saw the wind, he was afraid and, beginning to sink, cried out, "Lord, save me!" Immediately Jesus reached out his hand and caught him. "You of little faith," he said, "why did you doubt?"
—MATTHEW 14:25–31

WHEN JESUS TOLD Peter to come, Peter had a choice to make. He could either stay in the safety of the boat or participate in one of the most miraculous events in history. He got out of the boat even though he was scared. But then something happened: Peter took his eyes off Jesus and began to sink. Thankfully, Jesus rescued him. Yet He also challenged him to increase his faith. He calls us to do the same.

TAKE HEART

Would you get out of the boat? What is Jesus calling you to do now?

TAKE ACTION

Be bold. Follow the Lord's prompting. What is He calling you to do? You may have to step out of the safety of the boat and into the unknown.

Day 126
JUST A TOUCH

When they had crossed over, they landed at Gennesaret.
And when the men of that place recognized Jesus, they sent
word to all the surrounding country. People brought all their
sick to him and begged him to let the sick just touch the
edge of his cloak, and all who touched it were healed.
—MATTHEW 14:34–36

ONE OF MY favorite parts of the New Testament miracles is that the stories often say *all* were healed. I think many of us see Jesus as a kind of lottery where we might get lucky and win a miracle. Yet Jesus doesn't play games. He is God. In many of the miracle stories, we also see how the people desperately sought Jesus, with full faith He could heal them. It's not like swinging into the gas station and buying a Powerball ticket to see what happens. Jesus is a 100 percent guy. Are we bringing our full faith?

TAKE HEART

How have you viewed miracles or healing before? Do you see it as luck or a promise?

TAKE ACTION

If Jesus showed up right now in front of you and asked, "What do you want?" what would you say? Do it. He is here now.

Day 127
DO YOU HAVE A HEART CONDITION?

Jesus called the crowd to him and said, "Listen and understand. What goes into someone's mouth does not defile them, but what comes out of their mouth, that is what defiles them."
—MATTHEW 15:10–11

THERE IS MUCH confusion, opinion, and conflict around food. What's good? What's bad? But, as usual, Jesus has a different take. He's wondering about your heart. Jesus says, "Listen, food will come in and pass through you. That won't make you unclean, but your words show your heart." Mic drop.

Just think about how much time, money, resources, and thought people spend on food. Yet when it comes to our hearts and words, we too often hardly consider those. Jesus warns us big time. Let me put it this way: you could eat the cleanest diet in the world and still be the sickest, most unclean person.

TAKE HEART

Is your heart clean? How are the words coming out of your heart?

TAKE ACTION

Be extra intentional today about what comes out of your mouth. Imagine Jesus following you around all day (He is). What would He say?

PERSISTENCE PAYS

A Canaanite woman...came to [Jesus], crying out, "Lord, Son of David, have mercy on me! My daughter is demon-possessed and suffering terribly." Jesus did not answer a word....The woman came and knelt before him. "Lord, help me!" she said. He replied, "It is not right to take the children's bread and toss it to the dogs." "Yes it is, Lord," she said. "Even the dogs eat the crumbs that fall from their master's table." Then Jesus said to her, "Woman, you have great faith! Your request is granted." And her daughter was healed at that moment.
—MATTHEW 15:21–28

THIS INTERESTING MIRACLE shows us another facet of how we can relate with Jesus. Imagine if one of your children was really suffering—in this case, the daughter was demonized. This woman tracked down Jesus. She approached Him and asked Him to heal her daughter. Yet Jesus did not say a word to her! She kept asking, kept "bothering" Him. She pleaded her case. This woman was tenacious. Jesus then said, "You have great faith. Your request is granted." Her daughter was healed!

TAKE HEART

Think of something you prayed for. Did you quit when you didn't get the answer you needed right away?

TAKE ACTION

Be a relentless mama bear. What would have happened if this mother had stopped? She *knew* Jesus could heal her daughter. She wasn't going to stop asking Him.

GOD IS ENOUGH

Jesus left there and went along the Sea of Galilee. Then he went up on a mountainside and sat down. Great crowds came to him, bringing the lame, the blind, the crippled, the mute and many others, and laid them at his feet; and he healed them. The people were amazed when they saw the mute speaking, the crippled made well, the lame walking and the blind seeing. And they praised the God of Israel.
—MATTHEW 15:29–31

AGAIN, JESUS WAS on the move. People believed He could heal them, so they came to Him. Blind, crippled, lame, mute—He healed them all. Everyone was amazed. "And they *praised the God of Israel.*"

When Jesus heals you, it should lead you to praise Him. Miracles are incredible, but they are all intended to bring us to the Father. None of it matters without relationship with Him, without surrendering our lives to Him. It's like wanting only the stuff the Amazon guy gives you but not the person himself. We must be careful to know *who* the healer is and not just take from Him selfishly so we can get back to our lives. Many who were healed followed Jesus. They wanted to know more of Him.

TAKE HEART

Do you want God or just His benefits?

TAKE ACTION

Reflect and repent in an area you have been "using" God. He alone is enough.

Day 130

ANOTHER SUPERNATURAL BUFFET

*He told the crowd to sit down on the ground. Then he took
the seven loaves and the fish, and when he had given
thanks, he broke them and gave them to the disciples, and
they in turn to the people. They all ate and were satisfied. Afterward the disciples picked up seven basketfuls of
broken pieces that were left over. The number of those who
ate was four thousand men, besides women and children.*
—MATTHEW 15:35–38

I WONDER IF THE disciples ever got used to Jesus' miracles? We
can sometimes take for granted all the things He does for us
or even begin to feel entitled. Think about something as simple
as your heart beating. Jesus allows our hearts to beat. We hardly
even think about it. In this story, Jesus *fed over four thousand
people* with a few fish and loaves. And they were all satisfied!

Let us remain in *awe* of Jesus' wonder-working power,
from the simple breath we breathe, to the hanging of the stars,
to tremendous healings and other miracles. All miracles are
amazing, and they are around us every second.

TAKE HEART

There is a great quote that says, "There are only two ways to
live your life...as though nothing is a miracle...[or] as though
everything is a miracle." What way do you live?

TAKE ACTION

What are some miracles you have started to take for granted?
Write them down, and give thanks today.

Day 131
THINGS OF GOD OR THINGS OF MAN

But He turned and said to Peter, "Get behind Me, Satan!
You are an offense to Me, for you are not mindful of the
things that are of God, but those that are of men.
—MATTHEW 16:23, MEV

THE BRAIN IS better and faster than any supercomputer. It can store 2.5 million gigabytes of data and is estimated to process as fast as "a billion billion calculations per second."[1] It is smarter than any smartphone. We get so amazed by new technology, yet the most incredible tech ever created—*you*—is often taken for granted.

TAKE HEART

Do you take care of your brain? Do you feed it well, challenge it, and protect it?

TAKE ACTION

The brain needs to be challenged to stay sharp. Staring at TVs, phones, and computers and living on junk food and prescription drugs can affect brain function. Review your lifestyle as it relates to brain health. And *read*!

MOVE MOUNTAINS

A man...knelt before him. "Lord, have mercy on my son," he said. "He has seizures and is suffering greatly....I brought him to your disciples, but they could not heal him."...Jesus rebuked the demon, and it came out of the boy, and he was healed at that moment. Then the disciples...asked, "Why couldn't we drive it out?" He replied, "Because you have so little faith. Truly I tell you, if you have faith as small as a mustard seed, you can say to this mountain, 'Move from here to there,' and it will move. Nothing will be impossible for you."
—MATTHEW 17:14–20

DIFFERENT MIRACLES SHOW us different facets of Jesus and teach us something. In this case, a father with a demon-possessed son seeks out Jesus and the disciples for healing. The disciples try first, with no results. Next Jesus gets involved and effortlessly *heals the boy*. And then He busts the disciples' chops. He uses this teaching moment to challenge their faith. We must remember it is only through Christ that we can operate in these gifts. The minute we start to think we alone can do it or don't need faith or Jesus, we are finished.

TAKE HEART

Do you ever get prideful? Think you do things in your power, saying, "Look how hard I worked," etc.?

TAKE ACTION

List things that you have taken credit for. Repent and give the glory to God.

PROTECT OUR CHILDREN!

But whoever misleads one of these little ones who believe in Me, it would be better for him to have a millstone hung about his neck and to be drowned in the depth of the sea.
—MATTHEW 18:6, MEV

SOMETIMES PEOPLE ASK me why babies get sick or develop cancer. Now, of course, there are some things we will just never understand, but this is a critical issue we need to consider. Babies are now created in a toxic environment, even within the womb. Recent research has shown that the blood of birth moms often has hundreds of toxic and even cancer-causing chemicals in it.[1] We need to clean up the "fishbowl" so the "fish" can be healthy. Sometimes I am amazed we are not sicker!

TAKE HEART

The Bible discusses how important it is that we raise our children and protect them. Are we doing a good job of this? How can we improve?

TAKE ACTION

Unfortunately, our world is more toxic than ever, and we are learning more every day about the effects of these chemicals. Consider doing an annual or semiannual detox to keep yourself less toxic.

Day 134
WITH GOD *ALL* THINGS ARE POSSIBLE

*A man...asked, "Teacher, what good thing must I do to
get eternal life?" ...Jesus replied, "...If you want to enter
life, keep the commandments."..."All these I have kept," the
young man said. "What do I still lack?" Jesus answered, "...
Go, sell your possessions and give to the poor, and you
will have treasure in heaven. Then come, follow me." When
the young man heard this, he went away sad, because he
had great wealth. Then Jesus said to his disciples, "...It is
easier for a camel to go through the eye of a needle than for
someone who is rich to enter the kingdom of God." ...They...
asked, "Who then can be saved?" Jesus...said, "With man
this is impossible, but with God all things are possible."*
—MATTHEW 19:16–26

WE OFTEN QUOTE "With God all things are possible," but
we may forget the context. Jesus compared a rich man's
struggle to enter God's kingdom with a camel going through
the eye of a needle. The disciples said, "That's impossible!"
Jesus agreed, saying it was possible *only* with God—period.
We all need God. Money, fame, house, cars, career, social
media likes, and so on cannot get us into His kingdom.

TAKE HEART

Would you have responded differently than the young ruler?

TAKE ACTION

Reflect on your life. Where are you storing up treasure? List
two things to give away.

DESIGNED TO HEAL

TWO BLIND MEN—ANOTHER MIRACLE

Two blind men were sitting by the roadside, and when they heard that Jesus was going by, they shouted, "Lord, Son of David, have mercy on us!" The crowd rebuked them and told them to be quiet, but they shouted all the louder, "Lord, Son of David, have mercy on us!" Jesus stopped and called them. "What do you want me to do for you?" he asked. "Lord," they answered, "we want our sight." Jesus had compassion on them and touched their eyes. Immediately they received their sight and followed him.
—MATTHEW 20:30–34

JESUS WAS GETTING pretty popular. People were always gathered around Him. He was a bit of a big deal. In this instance, a couple of blind guys alongside the road called out to Jesus, asking for mercy. Annoyed, the people around them told them to be quiet. But the blind men shouted louder. Jesus stopped and asked what He could do for them. The men asked Him to restore their vision. Jesus healed them, and then…*they followed Him.* What a great lesson! Don't let others around you prevent you from calling out to the Lord.

TAKE HEART

Do you ever hide your faith because you are afraid of what others may think?

TAKE ACTION

Do something to show an outward expression of your faith. Pray publicly. Raise your hands in worship. Pray with your kids.

Day 136
FULL-FAITH PRAYERS

Seeing a fig tree by the road, [Jesus] went up to it but found nothing on it except leaves. Then he said to it, "May you never bear fruit again!" Immediately the tree withered. When the disciples saw this, they were amazed. "How did the fig tree wither so quickly?" they asked. Jesus replied, "Truly I tell you, if you have faith and do not doubt, not only can you do what was done to the fig tree, but also you can say to this mountain, 'Go, throw yourself into the sea,' and it will be done. If you believe, you will receive whatever you ask for in prayer."
—MATTHEW 21:19–22

PUT YOURSELF IN this scene. You're on a walk with Jesus. He sees a fruitless fig tree and curses it, and it immediately withers. You and all the others are amazed. But then Jesus says to you, "I'm telling you, if you have full faith, you can also do these things. You will receive whatever you ask for in prayer." What an amazing moment! Can you imagine? "Anything? *I* can move mountains? *What?*" Yet this is what the Lord said: "Have faith and do not doubt."

TAKE HEART

Do you struggle with doubt? Why? What if you were standing with Jesus in that moment? Would that change you?

TAKE ACTION

List areas where you feel you have full faith. List areas where you struggle with faith. Ask the Lord to increase your faith.

GOD'S DESIGN BEATS
MAN'S EVERY TIME

*Blind Pharisee! First clean the inside of the cup and
dish, and then the outside also will be clean.*
—MATTHEW 23:26

IMAGINE IF YOU could filter your blood through about two
million tiny filters—and if somehow you could fit those filters in an area about the size of your fists. That would be awesome! And wouldn't it be great if those filters did not need
batteries or electricity and if they worked around the clock?
Oh you do have these! They are your kidneys. *Thank You,
Jesus, for our kidneys and for cleaning us from the inside out!*

TAKE HEART

Have you ever done a detox? Your body is constantly detoxing,
better than any pill or supplement ever can.

TAKE ACTION

Drink half your body weight in ounces of water today. This
will help your body detox and support the God-given detox
power within!

GET TO THE CAUSE

Woe to you, scribes and Pharisees, hypocrites! You are like whitewashed tombs, which indeed appear beautiful outwardly, but inside are full of dead men's bones and of all uncleanness.
—MATTHEW 23:27, MEV

T HE INHERENT PROBLEM is that most pharmacologic strategies do not address the underlying causes of ill health in Western countries, which are not drug deficiencies," said Dr. Walter C. Willett, professor of epidemiology and nutrition at Harvard's School of Public Health.[1] I could not agree with this statement more. If we as a body of believers could simply understand this basic truth, we would all be so much better off. But due to marketing, ignorance, fear, and addiction, we simply ignore this truth and live in some form of delusion.

TAKE HEART

Why do you think we in the church are just as sick and medicated as those outside it? Why do you think most people don't even know the basic truth of Dr. Willett's statement?

TAKE ACTION

Once we know the truth, we are obligated to share it with others. Choose one or two people you care about, and share this information with them.

Day 139
BUT SOME DOUBTED

Then the eleven disciples went to Galilee, to the mountain where Jesus had told them to go. When they saw him, they worshiped him; but some doubted.
—Matthew 28:16–17

IMAGINE THAT YOU were at the last supper with Jesus, experienced all the events of the passion week, had seen all of His ministry, and now were seeing the resurrected Christ. Even with all that, the Bible says, "Some doubted." I have asked myself before if I would have been one of the doubters. But here is an important thing to remember: We don't create or muster up our faith. Our faith comes from God. It's a gift. We cannot increase our faith; only God does that.

Any faith that you have comes from God. Be thankful for any measure of faith He gave you. And pray and yearn that He increases your faith so your life can glorify Him even more!

TAKE HEART

Has God given you a strong measure of faith? Do you exercise your faith? Do you use it to bless others?

TAKE ACTION

Exercise or activate your faith. Look for opportunities today to engage your faith—maybe for a friend or a loved one.

Day 140

MORE HARM THAN GOOD?

She had suffered a great deal under the care
of many doctors and had spent all she had, yet
instead of getting better she grew worse.
—Mark 5:26

Accoding to a *British Medical Journal* article, the three leading causes of death in America are heart disease, cancer, and medical care.[1] This is a sobering and surprising statistic for many people. Several studies over the last couple decades continue to show that our health-care system is actually a leading cause of death. It is hard to understand how this can happen, but let me do my best to simplify it.

God created an infinitely complicated body. When we put pills, synthetic chemicals, and dangerous surgeries into or on it, there are often unforeseen consequences. Pride and arrogance with regard to "treating" our God-given bodies keep us from acknowledging that some things have not gone as planned. Our best bet for good health is not more drugs and surgeries; it is caring for and stewarding what God gave us.

Take Heart

Does this surprise you? Why? What does it make you want to change or reconsider? Are you more reliant on man's health care than God's care?

Take Action

We are called to steward our bodies. They are temples of the Holy Spirit. Do not hand your health over to someone else.

Day 141
EVEN JESUS ENJOYED EXERCISE—
HE WALKED ON WATER!

He saw the disciples straining at the oars, because
the wind was against them. Shortly before dawn
he went out to them, walking on the lake.
—MARK 6:48

IF EXERCISE COULD be packed into a pill, it would be the single most widely prescribed, and beneficial, medicine in the nation," said Dr. Robert Butler, founder of the National Institute on Aging.[1] This is another excellent quote to consider. When we truly understand the benefits God offers us when we exercise, we can see what a privilege it is to be able to move the bodies He gave us. We often spend more time complaining about this incredible gift than actually doing it! Exercise can be a form of worship to God, thanking Him for the body He created.

TAKE HEART

We need to reframe exercise from some painful, boring thing to the gift from God that it is. How do you see it?

TAKE ACTION

Do you exercise three to five times a week for twenty to thirty minutes? If not, now is the time!

Day 142

BE HONEST WITH JESUS—HE KNOWS ALREADY ANYWAY!

He took the blind man by the hand and led him outside the village. When he had spit on the man's eyes and put his hands on him, Jesus asked, "Do you see anything?" He looked up and said, "I see people; they look like trees walking around." Once more Jesus put his hands on the man's eyes. Then his eyes were opened, his sight was restored, and he saw everything clearly.
—MARK 8:23–25

ALTHOUGH JOHN 21:25 says all the world's books could not contain the stories of Jesus' miracles, I love the variety of His methods. He had no formula. But this was unique. Jesus spat on a blind man's eyes and laid His hands on him. When Jesus asked if he could see anything, the blind man said he could—but just a little bit. So Jesus laid hands on him again. This time, his eyes were fully opened.

Why twice? Why did Jesus not fully heal the blind man the first time? Why did Jesus ask whether he could see? Consider this: Jesus wants only the truth. When He asks us a question, we respond with *truth*. I bet many would have said, "Yep, it's better. Thanks!" and missed the *rest* of what Jesus wanted to do. He's a God of *all the way*. We need to just be honest.

TAKE HEART

Are you honest with Jesus?

TAKE ACTION

Pray right now, and no sugarcoating!

DESIGNED TO HEAL

Day 143
THE HEALING POWER OF SPIT

*He took the blind man by the hand and led him outside
the village. When he had spit on the man's eyes and put
his hands on him, Jesus asked, "Do you see anything?"*
—MARK 8:23

THE LIFESAVING, MIRACLE-WORKING, healing power of spit! Yes, your saliva serves a purpose. If you didn't make enough spit, you would not be able to digest food. *Thank You, Jesus, for* spit! If we didn't make spit every day, our mouths would become overrun with bacteria as well. Your body makes up to 1.5 liters of saliva each day! Hallelujah!

TAKE HEART

Our bodies are more than just parts and pieces. We are not a car. We are a dynamic, divine, self-healing, self-regulating creation. When is the last time you thought about that?

TAKE ACTION

Go outside and spit on the ground. Now give God thanks for spit. Your life depends on it!

THE BUTTERFLY

*Jesus took Peter, James, and John with him and
led them up a high mountain, where they were all
alone. There he was transfigured before them.*
—MARK 9:2

SOMETIMES GOD'S DESIGN just blows me away. Just consider
this: At some point a caterpillar decides all on its own to
create a chrysalis (cocoon). The caterpillar then basically liq-
uefies and turns into a kind of soup inside the chrysalis. Then
it reorganizes into a butterfly. Just think about that. How
much more intricately did God make you?

TAKE HEART

Isn't God's design amazing? And how much more amazing
are you?

TAKE ACTION

Today, be intentional about noticing and observing God's
design and world. Look at the trees, the sky, the birds, the
lake or ocean, the mountains. Just take it all in. Be in awe!

Day 145
LOVE

"Well said, teacher," the man replied. "You are right in saying that God is one and there is no other but him. To love him with all your heart, with all your understanding and with all your strength, and to love your neighbor as yourself is more important than all burnt offerings and sacrifices." When Jesus saw that he had answered wisely, he said to him, "You are not far from the kingdom of God."
—MARK 12:32–34

WHEN JESUS TEACHES about love, it's always a mic-drop moment. This time is no different. After Jesus explains that loving God and loving our neighbors are the greatest commandments, one of his listeners recognizes that this kind of love is more important than all the burnt offerings.

Folks, if you are struggling, trying to do everything right, know that *love* trumps it all. We can so easily slip into the bondage of religion and works and forget about love—unconditional love. Jesus will partner with you and ask you to walk this out with Him, but it all comes from love with Him!

TAKE HEART

Do your actions, behaviors, thoughts, and words come from a place of love? What about your self-talk?

TAKE ACTION

Today, start with love. Be intentional about how you speak, think, and act. Be like Jesus, Christian.

Day 146

WAKE UP—THE TRUTH IS
RIGHT IN FRONT OF YOU!

*Later Jesus appeared to the Eleven as they were eating; he
rebuked them for their lack of faith and their stubborn refusal
to believe those who had seen him after he had risen.*
—MARK 16:14

READING SCRIPTURE IS amazing. Some of the stories blow
me away, make me laugh, make me cry, or all of the above.
This one makes me think. So, Jesus was killed on the cross.
He told His disciples what was going to happen, but they
didn't get it. Think about this: they followed Jesus for three
years, saw countless miracles, and had many conversations all
day. Even still, they struggled. Jesus rose from the dead and
was appearing to people. This time He specifically appeared
to the eleven disciples, and what did He do? Rebuked them
for their lack of faith! Amazing. He was still trying to drive
home to them the importance of their faith. The risen Christ
stood right in front of the disciples, yelling, "Wake up, fellas!
It's time to get to work."

TAKE HEART

How would you have responded to seeing Jesus? Do you
struggle with unbelief?

TAKE ACTION

Read the last part of each of the four Gospels, and notice all
the ways Jesus showed up to the disciples.

LEAP FOR JOY

*Mary...entered Zechariah's home and greeted Elizabeth.
When Elizabeth heard Mary's greeting, the baby leaped
in her womb, and Elizabeth was filled with the Holy
Spirit. In a loud voice she exclaimed: "Blessed are you
among women, and blessed is the child you will bear!...As
soon as the sound of your greeting reached my ears, the
baby in my womb leaped for joy. Blessed is she who has
believed that the Lord would fulfill his promises to her!"*
—LUKE 1:39–45

ISN'T IT AMAZING how the presence of the Lord and being filled with the Holy Spirit can instantly change us? If you struggle with being stressed out, anxious, depressed, etc., know that the Holy Spirit loves to bring joy.

John the Baptist's mom, Elizabeth, and Jesus' mom, Mary, were related, possibly cousins. They were both pregnant at the same time. When they got together, John leaped for joy in Elizabeth's womb! What a great reminder of what happens when Jesus shows up! Here is the good news: if you have surrendered your life to Jesus, He not only shows up; He's inside you!

TAKE HEART

Does the presence of Jesus bring you joy?

TAKE ACTION

If you struggle with joy, the Lord is ready to help. Pray specifically for His presence, and also find a local church or another gathering of people who experience it.

HOW MANY GERMS DO YOU THINK WERE IN THE MANGER?

She gave birth to her firstborn, a son. She wrapped
him in cloths and laid him in a manger, because
there was no guest room available for them.
—Luke 2:7

THE IMMUNE SYSTEM God gave each of us is one of the most amazing things ever created. We still have only a very basic understanding of the complexities and the workings of the human body. Our immune systems are comprised of many different organisms.

All of our immune systems and body cells are integrated together by our brains and nerves. It is funny how much people worry about germs, considering how incredible the immune system is. The reality is, we are designed to live in harmony with our environment, and part of that is being exposed to the different things in our environment.

TAKE HEART

When you think of your immune system, what comes to mind? Do you have more *faith* in your immune system from God or *fear* of germs?

TAKE ACTION

Your lymph system (a part of your immune system) requires movement and water to process toxins. Drink a big glass of water, and take a walk!

Day 149
REJECTED

He went to Nazareth, where he had been brought up....He...
stood up to read...."The Spirit of the Lord is on me, because he
has anointed me." ...The eyes of everyone in the synagogue
were fastened on him. He [said], "Today this scripture is ful-
filled in your hearing." All spoke well of him...."Isn't this Joseph's
son?" they asked. Jesus said to them, "...Truly I tell you...no
prophet is accepted in his hometown....There were many in
Israel with leprosy in the time of Elisha the prophet, yet not
one of them was cleansed—only Naaman the Syrian." All the
people in the synagogue were furious when they heard this.
—Luke 4:16–28

As Christians we can be mocked, accused, persecuted, and, in some cases, killed. Jesus dealt with all this and said we would too. But it especially hurts when it comes from those closest to us. When Jesus returned to His hometown, the people grew upset, mocked Him, and threw Him out of town. In fact, they wanted to throw Him off a cliff! Not quite the "hometown hero"! But Jesus wasn't surprised. He did not let their attitude affect what He was called to do.

Take Heart

How do you respond when you are treated poorly because of your faith? Or do you keep silent, fearing what others may think, say, or do? What would Jesus say?

Take Action

Be bold. If they rejected Jesus, many will likely reject you!

Day 150
BREAK THE NETS!

[Jesus] said to Simon, "Put out into deep water, and let
down the nets for a catch." Simon answered, "Master, we've
worked hard all night and haven't caught anything. But
because you say so, I will let down the nets." When they
had done so, they caught such a large number of fish that
their nets began to break. So...[their partners] came and
filled both boats so full that they began to sink. When Simon
Peter saw this, he fell at Jesus' knees and said, "Go away
from me, Lord; I am a sinful man!"...Then Jesus said to Simon,
"Don't be afraid; from now on you will fish for people."
—LUKE 5:3–10

AFTER A BAD day of fishing, Jesus instructed Simon to put out the nets again. Simon was tired and frustrated and responded only out of obedience. To his surprise, the net got so full it began to break. In this moment, Simon was overwhelmed by Jesus. He immediately repented and felt unworthy to be in the Lord's presence.

Are you in a season where nothing seems to be working? Just keep doing what Jesus says! Be obedient. Cast out the nets, and expect a large catch. Jesus is faithful, even when we fall and fail and are tired and frustrated. Just do what He says.

TAKE HEART

Would you consider yourself obedient to Christ?

TAKE ACTION

What is something you know you should be doing? Do it today!

SOMETIMES YOU HAVE TO CUT A HOLE IN THE ROOF!

Some men came carrying a paralyzed man on a mat and tried to take him into the house to lay him before Jesus. When they could not find a way to do this because of the crowd, they went up on the roof and lowered him on his mat through the tiles into the middle of the crowd, right in front of Jesus.
—LUKE 5:18–19

WE'VE READ ABOUT this paralyzed man being healed before, in Matthew 9. But Luke provides another detail. He says that when the friends brought the paralytic to be healed by Jesus, the house was too crowded. So guess what these friends did? They cut a hole in the roof and lowered their paralytic friend down, *right in front of Jesus.* Man, those are some good friends. They found a way to get *front and center* with Jesus. You may need a little help from friends like these.

TAKE HEART

Do you have friends like that? Are you that kind of friend?

TAKE ACTION

Go out of your way to help a friend today.

NEW (WINE)SKINS

And no one pours new wine into old wineskins.
Otherwise, the new wine will burst the skins; the wine
will run out and the wineskins will be ruined.
—LUKE 5:37

SKIN IS A far more complicated organ than we often consider. Your skin defends against toxins and helps control your body's temperature. It is protective, but it also absorbs. What you put on yourself gets inside you.

This is such a good metaphor for life. We can often be contaminated by the things of the world by just being around them and absorbing them. We can get poisoned slowly and not even realize it.

TAKE HEART

What things of this world may be seeping into your heart? What or whom do you need to stop putting yourself around?

TAKE ACTION

In a very practical sense, you may be poisoning your body with chemicals and household or personal-use products. Do an audit of your home and the products you use.

Day 153
YOU CAN TELL A TREE BY ITS FRUIT

A good tree does not bear corrupt fruit, nor does a corrupt tree bear good fruit. Each tree is known by its own fruit....A good man out of the good treasure of his heart bears what is good, and an evil man out of the evil treasure of his heart bears what is evil.
—LUKE 6:43-45, MEV

IN THE UNITED States, spending on prescription drugs increased more than tenfold between 1980 and 2018.[1] Meanwhile, the health of the population has steadily declined.

This may be a surprising statistic, but just think about it logically for a moment. Even though we continue to consume more and more medications, we are not seeing improvements in our health. If the drugs were so helpful, wouldn't we be *healthier*? Hmm. This exposes a foundational assumption present in so much of our health care, and we need to be honest and reflect on this. We cannot drug ourselves to health. We must take responsibility for our actions and stop taking every pill we can find.

TAKE HEART

Why do you think we consume so many medications yet keep getting sicker? Do you research the drugs prescribed to you and decide whether to take them or blindly trust the doctor?

TAKE ACTION

See what your friends and family members think about this issue and how many medications they take.

Day 154
IT IS NEVER TOO LATE

*As [Jesus] approached the town gate, a dead person was being
carried out—the only son of his mother, and she was a widow....
When the Lord saw her, his heart went out to her and he said,
"Don't cry." Then he went up and touched the bier they were
carrying him on, and the bearers stood still. He said, "Young
man, I say to you, get up!" The dead man sat up and began
to talk....They were all filled with awe and praised God.*
—LUKE 7:12–16

A NOTHER INCREDIBLE MIRACLE from Jesus. As He came
into town, He saw a crowd of people surrounding a
coffin. A poor widow had lost her only son. It says when Jesus
saw her, His heart went out to her. Telling her not to cry, He
touched the coffin and told the young man to get up—*and he
did*. Amazing!

That's our God. He raises the dead from coffins. If He can
do that, I'm sure He can handle what you are going through.
What's fascinating is that the widow never asked for the miracle. Jesus did it out of compassion. Our Lord will do whatever He wants, whenever He wants, to whomever He wants.

TAKE HEART

What do you think of this story? Is it hard to believe? Do you
think resurrections still happen?

TAKE ACTION

He's the God of miracles, and it's never too late. Resurrect
some dreams and pray. Ask God to expand your faith.

CAN YOU WAIT JUST A SECOND, JESUS?

*Another said, "I will follow you, Lord; but first let
me go back and say goodbye to my family." Jesus
replied, "No one who puts a hand to the plow and
looks back is fit for service in the kingdom of God."*
—LUKE 9:61–62

THIS STORY HAS always fascinated me. Jesus is walking and
ministering, and people are captivated and deeply moved.
Some of them want to follow Him. Jesus tries to talk them out
of it, but a few are still committed to leaving it all to be His
disciples. But when one man wants to go say goodbye to his
family quick, Jesus rebukes him. Basically, Jesus tells him that
he doesn't really have what it takes.

This is some tough teaching. In today's standards we would
celebrate this man, throw a party for him, bring him on stage,
make a video about him, etc. However, Jesus would say, "You
don't have what it takes." Ouch.

TAKE HEART

Do you love Jesus more than anything? More than your kids?
Your family?

TAKE ACTION

Is there something Jesus has called you to that you are putting
off? Take a step toward doing it.

Day 156
DON'T MISS HIM

*A woman named Martha opened her home to him. She had
a sister called Mary, who sat at the Lord's feet listening to
what he said. But Martha was distracted by all the prepara-
tions that had to be made. She came to him and asked, "Lord,
don't you care that my sister has left me to do the work by
myself? Tell her to help me!" "Martha, Martha," the Lord
answered, "you are worried and upset about many things,
but few things are needed—or indeed only one. Mary has
chosen what is better, and it will not be taken away from her."*
—LUKE 10:38–42

IN TODAY'S FAST-PACED culture, it is so easy to become distracted—even when we're doing good things for Jesus. But
this story teaches us to slow down and just be with Jesus.

Martha welcomes Jesus into her home but is busy, stressed,
and distracted while He is there. Meanwhile, her sister, Mary,
just sits at Jesus' feet, doing nothing to help. Martha is so irri-
tated that she actually brings it up to Jesus. It's like when we
tell Jesus all the things we are doing for Him. He just says to
Martha, "Mary has chosen what is better." Just be with Jesus.

TAKE HEART

Are you a Martha or a Mary? Are you so busy you would miss
Jesus in front of you?

TAKE ACTION

Develop a habit of just being with the Lord. No agenda. No
distractions. He is enough.

DESIGNED TO HEAL

THE POWER OF PRAYER

One day Jesus was praying in a certain place. When he fin-ished, one of his disciples said to him, "Lord, teach us to pray, just as John taught his disciples." He said to them, "When you pray, say: 'Father, hallowed be your name, your kingdom come. Give us each day our daily bread. Forgive us our sins, for we also forgive everyone who sins against us. And lead us not into temptation.' ...If you then, though you are evil, know how to give good gifts to your children, how much more will your Father in heaven give the Holy Spirit to those who ask him!"
—LUKE 11:1–4, 13

IMAGINE BEING TAUGHT by Jesus how to pray. After seeing Jesus pray a lot, the disciples finally ask Him how to do it. So He teaches them this prayer. Amazing! Then He discusses the power of prayer and the goodness of God. He explains how, as loving parents, we always want to give our children the best we can. We would not give them a stone or snake if they asked for bread. And how much more does our perfect heavenly Father love us? This should give you incredible confidence and faith as you pray.

TAKE HEART

Did you have a good earthly father? Do you feel that God is a good father?

TAKE ACTION

Read and recite the Lord's Prayer. You are actually saying the words Jesus taught to the disciples. Wow!

THE EYE GATE

*Your eye is the lamp of your body. When your eyes are
healthy, your whole body also is full of light. But when
they are unhealthy, your body also is full of darkness.*
—LUKE 11:34

SEVERAL STUDIES HAVE shown that use of technology, social
media, and video games leads to increases in depression,
anxiety, isolation, and even obesity. Every year screen time
increases, and we are in worse shape for it. We have replaced
human interaction with some virtual version, and with meta-
verse looming, it will likely only get worse. The implications
are scary.

God designed us for relationship with Him and others.
Nothing can replace that.

TAKE HEART

How much time are you on screens? How about your kids and
grandkids? What effects are you seeing?

TAKE ACTION

Take a tech break. Lock it up, and log out. Get off for a season.
You won't regret it.

Day 159
FRANKENFOOD

Jesus began to speak first to his disciples, saying, "Be on your guard against the yeast of the Pharisees, which is hypocrisy."
—LUKE 12:1

HYDROGENATED SOYBEAN OIL, bleached wheat flour, aluminum phosphate, sodium acid pyrophosphate—those are just some of the ingredients in a McDonald's chicken nugget. As you struggle to pronounce things like these, I imagine you can see why eating these foods regularly (or even occasionally) can wreak havoc on your body and health. I often meet with parents who say things like "It is all my kids will eat." It is important we get educated about the ingredients in these foods and their potential impacts on our bodies and then work toward better, God-honoring choices.

TAKE HEART

God created you for more than this. Our bodies are not designed for these chemical concoctions. What do you think God thinks about these foods?

TAKE ACTION

Ignorance is not bliss—it's deadly. With the way things are in today's world, it is critical you learn about what is in food and how ingredients and chemicals can affect your health. Focus on eating food created by God, not food produced by man.

Day 160

YOU ARE MORE VALUABLE
THAN THE SPARROWS

*Indeed, even the hairs of your head are all numbered. Therefore
do not fear. You are more valuable than many sparrows.*
—Luke 12:7, MEV

THIS SCRIPTURE REMINDS us that God knows the number
of hairs on each of our heads. That is how personal and
specific our God is. Consider the billions of people on the
planet now and the billions who have lived before us. He
knows how many hairs all of us have had! On average, each
person's head has about one hundred thousand hairs—think
about that math!

Let this truth encourage you today. As you comb or brush
your hair, be reminded that God knows exactly how many
hairs you have. He knows more about you than *you* do!

TAKE HEART

How does it make you feel that God is a *specific* God? A personal God? He knows and cares about the details of your life.

TAKE ACTION

If God cares about the hairs on your head, He cares about
everything. What have you put off talking to Him about,
thinking He wouldn't care? Now would be a good time to
have that conversation.

Day 161
DO YOU REALLY NEED THAT SODA?

*Then he said to them, "Watch out! Be on your
guard against all kinds of greed; life does not con-
sist in an abundance of possessions."*
—Luke 12:15

SODA. POP. COLA. Isn't it ironic that when we want to "treat"
ourselves, we often eat or drink something that is actually
bad for our health. We might say, "Well, it's my only vice," or,
"It's my one treat of the day." Now, I am not here to shame you.
Drinking soda is not a sin. But it is important we know what
cola does to us. The chemicals, sugars, caffeine, acids, artificial colors, and so on mess up our God-given biology. It may
only be a can here or there, but just know it has effects.

Take Heart

Are you a soda drinker? Juice drinker? Could you quit?

Take Action

Stop drinking soda for twenty-one days. Replace it with carbonated water. You will be amazed at what this simple change
can do.

Day 162

MUCH IS ASKED

*From everyone who has been given much, much
will be demanded; and from the one who has been
entrusted with much, much more will be asked.*
—LUKE 12:48

I ONCE READ A great quote by a doctor in Ohio: "We have had amazing advances in the care we can provide as medical professionals, but the best medicine is prevention via a healthy lifestyle."[1] We often find ourselves waiting for man (creation) to figure out the ways of God (creator). Let this be a reminder that the greatest focus on health and healing is simply taking care of what God has given us already.

TAKE HEART

Do you find yourself waiting for the next pill or technology instead of caring for yourself?

TAKE ACTION

Pick one area of your lifestyle or habit you want to address. Maybe it is to eat a healthier breakfast or to stop drinking soda. Pick one. Start today.

Day 163

JESUS SAW HER

On a Sabbath Jesus was teaching in one of the syna-
gogues, and a woman was there who had been crippled
by a spirit for eighteen years. She was bent over and could
not straighten up at all. When Jesus saw her, he called
her forward and said to her, "Woman, you are set free
from your infirmity." Then he put his hands on her, and
immediately she straightened up and praised God.
—LUKE 13:10–13

THIS IS ONE of my favorite miracles. When Jesus was teaching one day, He saw a woman who had been bent over for eighteen years. He cast out a spirit of infirmity, and she was healed. She immediately began to praise God!

There are a few reasons I love this miracle. First, the woman put herself in a position to have an encounter with Jesus. Second, "Jesus saw her" and called her forward. I imagine she had probably given up on being well after all those years, but Jesus hadn't. Third, she immediately praised God. She had a spirit of thankfulness. What a drastic turn of events for her and everyone in the room.

TAKE HEART

Are you putting yourself in a position to have an encounter with Jesus?

TAKE ACTION

Get in the game. Get out of your comfort zone! Go to a conference, listen to a new sermon, or read a new book.

Day 164
JESUS HEALS

One Sabbath, when Jesus went to eat in the house of a promi-
nent Pharisee, he was being carefully watched. There in front
of him was a man suffering from abnormal swelling of his
body. Jesus asked the Pharisees and experts in the law, "Is
it lawful to heal on the Sabbath or not?" But they remained
silent. So taking hold of the man, he healed him and sent him
on his way. Then he asked them, "If one of you has a child
or an ox that falls into a well on the Sabbath day, will you
not immediately pull it out?" And they had nothing to say.
—LUKE 14:1–6

THE PHARISEES WERE always trying to catch Jesus doing
something wrong. In their presence Jesus healed a man
of dropsy (a buildup of fluid in his body). He then challenged
the Pharisees, yet they had nothing to say.

I love Jesus. I love His bold, relentless love and power. He
didn't shy away from debate. He didn't avoid difficult conversations or situations. He went head-on, showing and teaching
us about the ways of God. Nothing and no one will stop the
ways of the Lord!

TAKE HEART

Do you think there is anything Jesus cannot do? Do you think
He is intimidated by today's version of Pharisees?

TAKE ACTION

Be bold today. Pray for a stranger. Tell someone what Jesus
has done in your life, even if it is on the Sabbath.

Day 165

COUNT THE COSTS

For who among you, intending to build a tower,
does not sit down first and count the cost to see
whether he has resources to complete it?
—LUKE 14:28, MEV

WHEN WE THINK about our lifestyle choices, we need to consider both the long-term and short-term effects. When we eat cheap food that makes us sick, it is no longer "cheap." Also understand that Big Pharma does not want us living healthy, clean lifestyles because that would be bad for their bottom line. Remember, we are in the world but not of the world. We are a set-apart people. We should look different and live differently.

TAKE HEART

Once you see the games played by certain industries, you can often avoid their ploys and traps. You are designed to heal. Focus on doing things that support God's design!

TAKE ACTION

Are you living clean? Are you going against Big Pharma's agenda? Take responsibility for your health and lifestyle choices.

Day 166
CLEANSE THE TEMPLE

*Then He entered the temple and began to drive out
those who sold and bought in it, saying to them, "It
is written, 'My house will be a house of prayer,'
but you have made it 'a den of thieves.'"*
—LUKE 19:45–46, MEV

IF JESUS WALKED the earth in the flesh today, do you think He would be concerned about some things? About some churches? Some things taught in schools? In what areas would He be flipping tables? Do you think He would have concerns about the health-care industry? Would He be bothered by how we care for the temples (bodies) He gave us? By all the sexualization and porn industries? Do you think He is bothered by our dependence on drugs and medications? Of course no one knows for sure what Jesus would or would not do, but it is important we reflect on the ways of the world we are living in and apply a scriptural understanding to them.

TAKE HEART

Why does it seem that good things get corrupted so often? Why do we, even as Christians, get sucked into these situations? What areas do you feel Jesus would struggle with most today?

TAKE ACTION

Have you become numb to the "money changers in the temple"? Have you found yourself just going along, saying, "That's just how it is"? What needs to change? Where have you allowed the house of prayer to become a den of robbers?

Day 167
JESUS HEALS AN EAR!

When Jesus' followers saw what was going to happen,
they said, "Lord, should we strike with our swords?" And
one of them struck the servant of the high priest, cut-
ting off his right ear. But Jesus answered, "No more of
this!" And he touched the man's ear and healed him.
—LUKE 22:49–51

THIS IS ANOTHER fascinating miracle, which happened while Jesus was being arrested in the garden. Peter, obviously upset, took his sword and cut off a soldier's ear. Jesus was not happy, telling Peter, "No more of this!" Then He healed the soldier.

Imagine this scene. I doubt this soldier who came to arrest Jesus believed Jesus was the Messiah. I doubt he was "saved" or had much faith. But the Lord healed him anyway. Now it doesn't say this, but I bet he believed in Jesus after this happened.

We must never put a box around how and when and who Jesus decides to touch. We just celebrate His grace and mercy.

TAKE HEART

Can Jesus heal an unbeliever? If so, does that feel fair or unfair to you?

TAKE ACTION

Scripture says, "While we were still sinners, Christ died for us" (Rom. 5:8) and "He first loved us" (1 John 4:19). It's that perfect love that allows us to come to Him. Tell Him thank you.

THE VEIL WAS TORN

It was now about noon, and darkness came over the whole land until three in the afternoon, for the sun stopped shining. And the curtain of the temple was torn in two.
—LUKE 23:44–45

As JESUS WAS dying for your and my sins on the cross, things got pretty crazy. The Gospel accounts say the earth shook violently, the sun stopped shining, people came up out of graves, and, perhaps most importantly, the thick veil in the temple (estimated to be several inches thick) was torn in two from top to bottom.

This veil separated man from God. Not just anyone could go behind it. Yet Jesus' death changed that. Now anyone could go directly to God. Amazing! Many who witnessed this event believed in Jesus afterward. Some who had been mocking and laughing now saw Him for who He was—the Messiah.

TAKE HEART

Do you go directly to God? Do you have a personal relationship with Him? Scripture says He knows how many hairs are on your head. Jesus went to the cross because and for you.

TAKE ACTION

You have direct access to God. Pray to Him right now, and thank Him for that.

Day 169
WATER INTO WINE

When the wine was gone, Jesus' mother said to him, "They have no more wine." "Woman, why do you involve me?" Jesus replied....His mother said to the servants, "Do whatever he tells you." Nearby stood six stone water jars...each holding from twenty to thirty gallons. Jesus said to the servants, "Fill the jars with water"; so they filled them to the brim. Then he told them, "Now draw some out and take it to the master of the banquet." They did so, and the master of the banquet tasted the water that had been turned into wine....Then he...said, "Everyone brings out the choice wine first...but you have saved the best till now."
—JOHN 2:3–10

DID YOU KNOW Jesus' first miracle was turning water into wine at a wedding? Here is the aspect of this I want to focus on: No one (besides Jesus' mom) knew Jesus could perform miracles. They were not demanding that He fix the party. They simply obeyed what He told them to do. Often we spend too much time trying to figure God out or asking Him for help instead of just being obedient to what He already said.

TAKE HEART

What does the word *obedience* bring to mind? Think about the opportunity to walk out God's design for you. How does that make you feel?

TAKE ACTION

List times you have obeyed God and times you haven't. How did that go?

"DO YOU WANT TO GET WELL?"

*There is in Jerusalem...a pool...called Bethesda....Here a great
number of disabled people used to lie—the blind, the lame, the
paralyzed. One who was there had been an invalid for thirty-
eight years. When Jesus saw him lying there...he asked him, "Do
you want to get well?" "Sir," the invalid replied, "I have no one
to help me into the pool when the water is stirred. While I am
trying to get in, someone else goes down ahead of me." Then
Jesus said to him, "Get up! Pick up your mat and walk." At
once the man was cured; he picked up his mat and walked.*
—JOHN 5:2–9

WHAT A POWERFUL scene. An invalid of thirty-eight years
was sitting by an area known for healing. Jesus heard
his story, then asked a somewhat strange question: "Do you
want to get well?" But instead of giving a quick and obvious
yes, the man gave Jesus an excuse of why he couldn't—that
it wasn't fair; he couldn't get to the healing waters. Have you
ever given Jesus excuses for why you cannot do something?
Well, Jesus told the man to get up and walk, and he was completely healed!

TAKE HEART

Why are we so good at making excuses, even to Jesus? I love
how Jesus just ignored the excuse and *spoke life*!

TAKE ACTION

Reflect on how you talk and think. Do you make a lot of
excuses? Take them to God. He's bigger than any excuse.

Day 171
HE IS THE BREAD OF LIFE

*Jesus answered, "...you are looking for me...because you
ate the loaves and had your fill. Do not work for food that
spoils, but for food that endures to eternal life, which the
Son of Man will give you...." ...Jesus said to them, "...For the
bread of God is the bread that comes down from heaven
and gives life to the world....I am the bread of life. Whoever
comes to me will never go hungry, and whoever believes in
me will never be thirsty....And whoever comes to me I will
never drive away....For my Father's will is that everyone who
looks to the Son and believes in him shall have eternal life."*
—JOHN 6:26–40

THIS IS A powerful passage. Of all that we could discuss
about it, here are a couple observations. First, we often
want the "stuff" from God—the healing, the free food—but
Jesus strongly reminds us it is about Him alone. He is the
bread of life, not just a good baker and doctor. Second, He
is the only way. We have to come and surrender our lives to
Him; He alone will save us.

This convicting passage reminds us to be mindful of why
we seek God. Do we want Him to be our Santa Claus, or do
we want Him and Him alone? He is our bread of life.

TAKE HEART

Is Jesus enough?

TAKE ACTION

Meditate on this passage. Ask God what He wants to show you.

Day 172
THE TRUTH HURTS

Many of his disciples said, "This is a hard teaching. Who can accept it?" ...Jesus said to them, "Does this offend you?...The Spirit gives life; the flesh counts for nothing. The words I have spoken to you...are full of the Spirit and life. Yet there are some of you who do not believe." ...He went on to say, "This is why I told you that no one can come to me unless the Father has enabled them." From this time many of his disciples turned back and no longer followed him. "You do not want to leave too, do you?" Jesus asked the Twelve. Simon Peter answered him, "Lord, to whom shall we go? You have the words of eternal life.
—JOHN 6:60–68

Jesus was doing some hard preaching, and some of His followers did not like it. What did Jesus say? "Does this offend you?" Oftentimes the truth hurts.

Jesus *spoke only truth*. If you don't like what Jesus is speaking, it's you who needs to adjust, not Him. Too much of today's preaching is watered down, "tickling the ears." In fact, it's almost a crime now to offend someone with the truth. Truth sounds like hate, to people who hate truth. When the teaching gets tough, stay in the game. Don't quit!

TAKE HEART

Does your church preach hard truths? How do you respond to some of the tougher teachings?

TAKE ACTION

Do you need to get uncomfortable? Is it time you found some stronger teaching? Try a small group or something similar.

Day 173
MY GLORY IS NOTHING

Jesus replied, "If I glorify myself, my glory
means nothing. My Father, whom you claim as
your God, is the one who glorifies me."
—JOHN 8:54

O H HOW WE love to glorify ourselves. "Look at me. Give
me attention. Like my social media posts. Make me feel
good and affirm me no matter what I do. Be nice." When you
know God and do what God commands you, Jesus promised
and prophesied that the world will hate you. Our culture wor-
ships celebrities of all types: athletes, actors, business leaders,
and even "celebrity" pastors. A 2019 survey found that 54 percent of kids want to be "social media influencers" and 86 percent are willing to try it at least once.[1]

This is not the way of the Lord. Such focus on self and
looks and likes has destroyed the hearts of many. We must
return our hearts fully to the Lord. Let us be able to say the
same words Jesus said and remember our glory is nothing.

TAKE HEART

It is hard to consider we care more about our cars, houses,
or sports teams than Jesus. But our actions, time, and energy
suggest otherwise. How are you doing in this area?

TAKE ACTION

Ask the Lord to show you where you are not glorifying Him.
Where are you self-glorifying, and what needs to change?

Day 174
FOR THE GLORY OF GOD

*As he went along, he saw a man blind from birth. His disciples
asked him, "Rabbi, who sinned, this man or his parents, that
he was born blind?" "Neither this man nor his parents sinned,"
said Jesus, "but this happened so that the works of God might
be displayed in him....." After saying this, he spit on the ground,
made some mud with the saliva, and put it on the man's eyes.
"Go," he told him, "wash in the Pool of Siloam" (this word means
"Sent"). So the man went and washed, and came home seeing.*
—JOHN 9:1–7

THIS IS ANOTHER powerful healing miracle that challenges
us. Jesus noticed a man who had been blind since birth.
Jesus told the disciples that the blindness wasn't to punish the
man or his parents for sin but to display "the works of God"
in his life. Then Jesus spit in some dirt, made mud, rubbed
it in the man's eyes, and gave him a couple of instructions,
which he followed and was healed! Amazing.

TAKE HEART

Have you ever considered that some struggles in your life and
others' lives are there purely to glorify God? Does that change
your perspective?

TAKE ACTION

It's not always sin, the devil, or someone else's fault. Sometimes
God shows up in areas and situations that surprise us. Be
open today to being surprised by Jesus. He still has much to
teach you!

GOD IS THE CREATOR OF LIFE!

The thief comes only to steal and kill and destroy; I have come that they may have life, and have it to the full.
—JOHN 10:10

YOU MAY HAVE seen the headlines: "U.S. life expectancy down; drug overdose, suicide up sharply."[1] When you read news like this, it is hard to not get really upset at the devil's plans. When we look at all the people addicted and overdosing on drugs and committing suicide, it exposes just how far from God's design and plans we have gone. We are destroying ourselves. As Hosea 4:6 reminds us, we "are destroyed from lack of knowledge." Jesus wants to give us life to the full.

TAKE HEART

When is enough, enough? When will we wake up to the lie that chasing this world has created? The stress of trying to get all the material things and chase the next high is literally killing us.

TAKE ACTION

We are reminded to be in this world, but not of this world. Reflect on your daily choices, the condition of your heart. Are you chasing the world?

Day 176
WHOM ARE YOU LISTENING TO?

My sheep hear My voice, and I know them, and they follow Me.
—JOHN 10:27, MEV

THE DEVIL IS a liar. He will use any trick he can to destroy you, but he has been defeated. When it comes to our lives and health, we can often fall for the tricks of the enemy. The devil's voice condemns, confuses, pushes, frightens, rushes, and worries us. But God's voice calms, comforts, convicts, encourages, enlightens, leads, reassures, and stills us.

TAKE HEART

Whose voice are you listening to?

TAKE ACTION

Choose an area where you have been listening to the enemy. Take it to God. Pray for protection from the enemy. Pray out loud. Bind the enemy's ways in Jesus' name.

LAZARUS, COME OUT

Jesus, once more deeply moved, came to the tomb.... "Take away the stone," he said. "But, Lord," said Martha, the sister of the dead man, "by this time there is a bad odor, for he has been there four days." Then Jesus said, "Did I not tell you that if you believe, you will see the glory of God?" So they took away the stone....Jesus called in a loud voice, "Lazarus, come out!" The dead man came out, his hands and feet wrapped with strips of linen, and a cloth around his face. Jesus said to them, "Take off the grave clothes and let him go."
—JOHN 11:38–44

I'M SURE YOU have heard the story of Jesus raising Lazarus from the dead. As we have seen, the Bible shares several stories of the dead coming to life. Yet they all eventually died again—even Lazarus. There is only one person who overcame death permanently, and that is Jesus. So my question in relation to this miracle is, *How are you going to live?* What are you going to do with the time God gave you? Do not waste your life!

TAKE HEART

When Lazarus came back to life, do you think his new perspective was better? More thankful?

TAKE ACTION

Get on with living! Pour out your life as a burnt offering. Don't just suck up oxygen. Use the gift God gave you to be a blessing to others.

Day 178
PEACE OF MY HEART

*Peace I leave with you; my peace I give you. I do
not give to you as the world gives. Do not let not
your hearts be troubled and do not be afraid.*
—JOHN 14:27

THE MOST COMMON time for heart attacks is Monday
morning![1] Why? Because often people are stressed by
work at the beginning of the week. So stress, not cholesterol
or chronic high blood pressure, is a leading cause of heart
attacks. (Or perhaps Mondays are just really dangerous.)

It is important to understand the role stress plays in your
life. The Scriptures talk about a peace that surpasses all
understanding (Phil. 4:7). We are promised that even though
we will have struggles, God will never forsake us (Heb. 13:5).

TAKE HEART

Your perspective of God has so much to do with the peace
you experience in life. "No God, no peace. Know God, know
peace."

TAKE ACTION

Are you at peace? Are you reading the Word? He is at the door
knocking. Will you let Him in?

THE VINE

I am the true vine, and my Father is the gardener. He cuts off every branch in me that bears no fruit, while every branch that does bear fruit he prunes so that it will be even more fruitful. You are already clean because of the word I have spoken to you. Remain in me, as I also remain in you. No branch can bear fruit by itself; it must remain in the vine. Neither can you bear fruit unless you remain in me.
—JOHN 15:1–4

HAVE YOU EVER broken a branch off a tree? For a while it seems fine—the leaves might still be green, and it may even look healthy and alive—but the reality is, it is dying. It's no longer connected to life. It will no longer bear fruit.

Jesus uses this metaphor to help us understand who He is and how we must remain and abide in Him to stay alive and fruitful. But sometimes we think we can do it without Him. We fool ourselves because we are disconnected from the vine. We think we are fine until we start to grow weary. Our "leaves" begin to wilt, and we realize we need Jesus.

TAKE HEART

Have you noticed this in your life? Do you get disconnected from the source? How has that worked for you?

TAKE ACTION

Reflect on your life. Where are you trying to do life without God? Focus on those areas. Resurrect and reconnect to God.

DON'T BURY YOUR HEAD IN THE SAND

Meanwhile Simon Peter was standing and warming himself. So they said to him, "Are you not also one of His disciples?" He denied it and said, "I am not!"
—JOHN 18:25, MEV

THE PROBLEM WITH many toxins and chemicals is that they are invisible. You can't smell or taste them, and they are impossible to see. So we often think we are not being affected, or when something goes wrong, we don't realize it could be from the toxins in or around us. We don't want to believe some of the things we do may be hurting us. Sometimes it seems easier to bury our heads in the sand. Ignorance is bliss, and maybe deadly. Thank God He built some pretty amazing detox systems into us, but the levels of chemicals and toxins we are now exposed to are so large that we need to be extra assertive.

TAKE HEART

Does this surprise you? Do you try to avoid toxic chemicals in your home, food, and personal-care products?

TAKE ACTION

Support natural body-detox methods. Drink lots of clean water daily, exercise, and use saunas, colonics, and other natural ways to help detox.

DOUBTING THOMAS

Thomas...was not with the disciples when Jesus came. So the other disciples told him, "We have seen the Lord!" But he said to them, "Unless I...put my finger where the nails were, and put my hand into his side, I will not believe." A week later...Thomas was with them. Though the doors were locked, Jesus came and stood among them and said, "Peace be with you!" Then he said to Thomas, "Put your finger here; see my hands. Reach out your hand and put it into my side. Stop doubting and believe." Thomas said to him, "My Lord and my God!" Then Jesus told him, "Because you have seen me, you have believed; blessed are those who have not seen and yet have believed."
—JOHN 20:24–29

HAVE YOU HEARD the term *doubting Thomas*? It comes from this disciple who was skeptical that Jesus had resurrected. He wouldn't believe it until he saw Jesus for himself. So Jesus showed up one day and had Thomas touch the wounds in His hands and side. Now Thomas believed! But here's the great part: Jesus then said, "Sure, you believe because you have seen, but blessed are those who believe and have *not seen*!"

TAKE HEART

Have you ever said, "If Jesus does ____, then I will believe"? What does Jesus say about that? Do you still doubt today?

TAKE ACTION

Faith is belief and trust in things unseen. Challenge yourself, and ask God to give you faith to believe without seeing.

FEED MY SHEEP

The third time he said to him, "Simon son of John, do you love me?" Peter was hurt because Jesus asked him the third time, "Do you love me?" He said, "Lord, you know all things; you know that I love you." Jesus said, "Feed my sheep.
—JOHN 21:17

EATING DOES NOT mean you are being fed or nourished. Your body is not built from calories; it is built from nutrition. When we are looking at what to eat or fuel our bodies with, what matters is nutrients, not calories. So make sure you are getting plenty of nutrition in your diet! Consider eating food as close as possible to how God designed it. Consuming plenty of vegetables, nuts, seeds, water, herbal tea, and clean and lean meats is a great start.

TAKE HEART

You are fearfully and wonderfully made. Your body is one of the most amazing creations God ever made. Give it what it is designed to have.

TAKE ACTION

This week, when you're eating or shopping, eat based on nutrients and not calories.

THE HOLY SPIRIT COMES

When the day of Pentecost came, they were all together in one place. Suddenly a sound like the blowing of a violent wind came from heaven and filled the whole house where they were sitting. They saw what seemed to be tongues of fire that separated and came to rest on each of them. All of them were filled with the Holy Spirit and began to speak in other tongues as the Spirit enabled them.
—Acts 2:1–4

THIS WAS A very important moment in history. As the disciples were all together in one place, the Holy Spirit came like a rushing wind and filled the house, and amazing things began to happen. They were now filled with the Holy Spirit. This had never happened before. Jesus had talked about this when He promised to send a helper who would live *in* His followers. Of course, the Holy Spirit has always existed, and at times He would rest on people. But this was a whole new ball game!

The promise of having the Holy Spirit in us is available to all believers—every one of us—and *it changes everything*! Get filled with the Holy Spirit!

TAKE HEART

Do you know you have the Holy Spirit in you? How?

TAKE ACTION

Imagine this moment. What has the Holy Spirit shown you? List Holy Spirit moments you have experienced.

HEALING IN THE NAME OF JESUS

A man who was lame from birth was being carried to the temple gate...to beg....When he saw Peter and John about to enter, he asked them for money....Then Peter said, "Look at us!" So the man gave them his attention....Then Peter said, "Silver or gold I do not have, but what I do have I give you. In the name of Jesus Christ of Nazareth, walk." Taking him by the right hand, he helped him up, and instantly the man's feet and ankles became strong. He jumped to his feet....Then he went with them into the temple courts, walking and jumping, and praising God.
—ACTS 3:2–8

THIS IS SUCH a powerful story. Now, remember, this is after Jesus was resurrected and the Holy Spirit filled the disciples. A man, crippled since birth, asks John and Peter for money. Peter says, "I don't have gold and silver, but in the name of Jesus of Nazareth, walk." Immediately, the man was healed! He followed them, walking, jumping, and praising God.

Here are just a few points to consider from this story: First, the man did not ask for healing. Jesus healed him. He went to the cause. Second, the man had been crippled since birth! Nothing is too hard for God. Finally, note that this healing happened through Spirit-filled believers.

TAKE HEART

Do you think you have the faith to speak like Peter and John?

TAKE ACTION

Pray for someone's healing, in Jesus' name, today.

OBEY GOD, NOT MAN

*Then they called them in again and commanded them not
to speak or teach at all in the name of Jesus. But Peter
and John replied, "Which is right in God's eyes: to listen
to you, or to him? You be the judges! As for us, we cannot
help speaking about what we have seen and heard.*
—ACTS 4:18–20

WHEN YOU BEGIN to operate as a Spirit-filled believer, not everyone will enjoy the change in you. Friends, family, coworkers, etc., may begin to be bothered.

After Peter and John healed the crippled man and were speaking about who Jesus is and what He came to do, the Sanhedrin (the religious leaders) were not happy. They tried to intimidate Peter and John, telling them they could no longer talk or teach about Jesus. But Peter and John replied that they could not stop speaking about what they had seen and heard. Now, remember, this is the *same Peter* who denied Christ three times. The disciples had a newfound boldness after the resurrection of Jesus and the outpouring of the Holy Spirit. They were *fearless*!

TAKE HEART

Are you more afraid of man or God? Be honest with yourself. What do you need to change?

TAKE ACTION

Speak up. Next time you are in a situation where it seems scary to share Jesus' truth, do it anyway! Share your testimony.

THE APOSTLES HEALED MANY

The apostles performed many signs and wonders among the people. And...more and more men and women believed in the Lord and were added to their number. As a result, people brought the sick into the streets and laid them on beds and mats so that at least Peter's shadow might fall on some of them as he passed by. Crowds gathered also from the towns around Jerusalem, bringing their sick and those tormented by impure spirits, and all of them were healed.
—ACTS 5:12–16

SOME PEOPLE STRUGGLE to believe that Jesus still heals today. I think you can answer this very simply: Does a cut on your arm heal? Do broken bones mend? You have somewhere between 37 and 100 trillion cells in your body; somehow they know what to do all together and all the time.

Yet what people often mean is, Does Jesus still heal miraculously? That answer is yes. This story talks about how crowds would gather around the area where the disciples were so they could be healed. People were carried there on beds and mats, and the scripture says, "All were healed." Praise the Lord!

TAKE HEART

Why do some find it so hard to believe in miracles? Is it hard for you? There are so many miraculous things around us.

TAKE ACTION

List miraculous things like babies, stars, oceans, our solar system, love, and so on. Let them blow your mind.

DO YOU BELIEVE IN MIRACLES?

*Now Stephen, full of faith and power, did great
wonders and miracles among the people.*
—ACTS 6:8, MEV

ONE OF THE most amazing miracles I have ever seen was in a patient who had a massive brain tumor. She likely got this tumor from living next to and working in a refinery for most of her life. Most doctors told her nothing could be done, but she found one surgeon willing to try. Still, they warned her that she would have *serious* loss of function after surgery—if she even survived. She survived the surgery. She has zero loss of function or memory. Incredible!

TAKE HEART

Do you believe in miracles? Have you seen one? Several?

TAKE ACTION

Seek out miracles. Pray for miracles. Talk to others about miracles they have seen or experienced. Miracles help encourage us and strengthen our faith.

SIT UP STRAIGHT!

*You stiff-necked people! Your hearts and ears are
still uncircumcised. You are just like your ances-
tors: You always resist the Holy Spirit!*
—ACTS 7:51

THE BIBLE NEVER speaks well of people with stiff necks. A spine is designed to move! Research has shown that losing three or more centimeters of height as they age can cause a 64 percent increase in heart-related deaths for men.[1] And other research has shown that the worse your overall posture, the worse your overall health.

Stand up straight! Remember when your mom or grandma chastised you for your posture? Well, they were right again! These studies show just how important our posture can be. With all the technology people have and the sedentary life-styles many lead, it is more important than ever to make sure we are caring for our spines and posture.

TAKE HEART

Do you pay attention to your posture? Do you do spinal stretches or exercises on a regular basis?

TAKE ACTION

Get your posture assessed by a person who is qualified to do that. A good structural or chiropractic exam is critical to caring for your frame!

STONED TO DEATH

*When...the Sanhedrin heard this, they were furious and
gnashed their teeth at him...."Look," [Stephen] said, "I see
heaven open and the Son of Man standing at the right hand
of God." At this they...dragged him out of the city and began
to stone him. Meanwhile, the witnesses laid their coats at the
feet of a young man named Saul. While they were stoning
him, Stephen prayed, "Lord Jesus, receive my spirit." Then
he fell on his knees and cried out, "Lord, do not hold this
sin against them." When he had said this, he fell asleep.*
—Acts 7:54–60

WHILE STEPHEN WAS being stoned to death, Saul (later Paul) was overseeing it. This amazing passage reminds us of several things. Even as we learn about God's miracles and healings, we know that all of us will die. When people witnessed Stephen's stoning, they were moved by his faith, and it is reported that many were saved after witnessing his death. Your life matters. Run the race God has called you to run! Our lives will each look different and unique. It may seem rough at times, but I assure you Stephen (and Paul) are doing just fine.

TAKE HEART

How would you respond in this type of situation? What would you do for Christ? Are you willing to *live* for Him?

TAKE ACTION

Are you afraid of death? Why? Write the reasons down, and then take them to God.

THERE WAS GREAT JOY IN THE CITY

*Those who had been scattered preached the word wher-
ever they went. Philip went down to a city in Samaria and
proclaimed the Messiah there. When the crowds heard
Philip and saw the signs he performed, they all paid close
attention to what he said. For with shrieks, impure spirits
came out of many, and many who were paralyzed or
lame were healed. So there was great joy in that city.*
—ACTS 8:4–8

AFTER STEPHEN'S DEATH, there was great persecution. Saul
(Paul) went door to door to imprison Christians. Many
believers scattered, but they preached the word wherever they
went! Philip went to Samaria, where demons were cast out
and many paralyzed and lame people were healed. Amazing!

Isn't it interesting how much paralysis was healed in the
Scriptures? It's considered impossible in today's medical model,
yet average, everyday Spirit-filled believers were doing it effortlessly. And mind you, this was just after their friend was murdered. Jesus can heal anyone, at any time, through anyone.

TAKE HEART

How do you respond to trauma or fear? What do you think
Jesus would tell you?

TAKE ACTION

Do you pray for miracles? Have you ever laid hands on
someone or prayed and asked for healing? Start today.

SAUL IS CHANGED

[Ananias] said, "Brother Saul, the Lord—Jesus, who appeared to you on the road as you were coming here—has sent me so that you may see again and be filled with the Holy Spirit." Immediately, something like scales fell from Saul's eyes, and he could see again. He got up and was baptized, and after taking some food, he regained his strength.... At once he began to preach in the synagogues that Jesus is the Son of God. All those who heard him were astonished.
—ACTS 9:15–21

I'M SURE YOU have heard about Saul's miraculous conversion. This story should encourage you no matter where you (or those you love) are in your faith walk. Saul was actively persecuting and murdering Christians. And then he had a dramatic encounter with the Lord that changed everything. His world was turned upside down.

You may have said a prayer ten or twenty years ago. You may go to church regularly. But is your relationship with the Lord *fresh*? Full of adventure? Are you regularly seeing the fruit of the Spirit in your life? Are you pressing in for it?

TAKE HEART

When is the last time you were overwhelmed by the presence of the Lord?

TAKE ACTION

Get quiet and ask the Lord for a fresh touch. Or get outside your comfort zone and go to a revival or evangelistic meeting.

Day 192
ROLL UP YOUR MAT

As Peter traveled about the country, he went to visit the Lord's people who lived in Lydda. There he found a man named Aeneas, who was paralyzed and had been bedridden for eight years. "Aeneas," Peter said to him, "Jesus Christ heals you. Get up and roll up your mat." Immediately Aeneas got up. All those who lived in Lydda and Sharon saw him and turned to the Lord.
—ACTS 9:32–35

O NE REASON I wrote this book was to overwhelm you with the wonder-working power of God from the beginning of the Scriptures to the end. The sheer magnitude and spectrum of healings and restorations are amazing. This is no exception. This is another straightforward, extraordinary miracle. A man named Aeneas had been bedridden and paralyzed for eight years. Did you read that? Eight years! Peter said to him, "Jesus Christ heals you. Rise and make your bed." And he did! Mic drop.

Are there people who can speak into your life like this? Do you speak like this to others? To yourself? What would happen if you did?

TAKE HEART

What do you think about all these healing miracles in the Scriptures?

TAKE ACTION

Right now, in the name of Jesus, pray for someone's healing—either for someone you can think of or for yourself!

ANOTHER RESURRECTION

A disciple named Tabitha ([or] Dorcas)...was always doing good and helping the poor. About that time she became sick and died....[The disciples] sent two men to [Peter] and urged him, "Please come at once!" Peter went with them....All the widows stood around him, crying....Peter sent them all out of the room; then he got down on his knees and prayed. Turning toward the dead woman, he said, "Tabitha, get up." She opened her eyes, and seeing Peter she sat up. He took her by the hand and helped her to her feet. Then he called for the believers...and presented her to them alive. This became known all over Joppa, and many people believed in the Lord.
—ACTS 9:36–42

TRY TO PUT yourself in this scenario. A wonderful, godly woman who had done many good, compassionate works passed away. When her friends heard Peter was in a nearby town, they sent for him. Peter then knelt by her body and prayed. She opened her eyes and sat up. This became known all throughout the area, and because of that, many believed in the Lord! Signs, wonders, and miracles increase people's faith and stir belief. I pray that these stories do the same for you today.

TAKE HEART

Have you ever considered how God doing a miracle in your life could increase others' faith?

TAKE ACTION

Have you had a miracle or seen a miracle? Tell someone!

YOU'VE GOT THIS!

*So after they had fasted and prayed, they placed
their hands on them and sent them off.*
—Acts 13:3

HERE IS SOME more good news about fasting! If you are fasting *and* you exercise, you get two times the fat burn.[1] If you are trying to lose weight and gain muscle, this is a great habit to include.

TAKE HEART

Can you imagine fasting *and* exercising? You've got this!

TAKE ACTION

Pick a day to try this. You may be surprised how well you do and feel! Write down the challenges and victories.

EVEN IN PRISON

Paul and Silas were praying and singing hymns to God, and the other prisoners were listening to them. Suddenly there was such a violent earthquake that the foundations of the prison were shaken. At once all the prison doors flew open, and everyone's chains came loose. The jailer...was about to kill himself....But Paul shouted, "Don't harm yourself! We are all here!" The jailer...brought them out and asked, "Sirs, what must I do to be saved?" They replied, "Believe in the Lord Jesus, and you will be saved—you and your house-hold."...The jailer...was filled with joy because he had come to believe in God—he and his whole household.
—ACTS 16:25–34

W E'VE ALL PROBABLY felt stuck or at our wits' end. It's often hard to worship and give glory to God in these situations. Paul and Silas were in prison, yet they were singing and worshipping God. Then an earthquake set them free. The guard was so moved by what happened that he asked, "What must I do to be saved?" Paul said, "Believe in the Lord Jesus." The guard and all his family believed and were baptized. So even when you are in a bad way or place, consider that the Lord may be using it to minister to others. It's not about you!

TAKE HEART

Do you find it hard to glorify God in tough times?

TAKE ACTION

If you're struggling in an area, try praising God. It changes you.

Day 196
MOVE!

For in him we live and move and have our being.
—ACTS 17:28

MOVEMENT IS POWERFUL. God designed us to be a people who move. Everything with life moves. The more we move, the more alive we feel.

There are so many amazing benefits of exercise and movement, but here is one of the best: research shows that the more you move, the lower your chance of developing thirteen different types of cancer![1] You can literally run away from cancer!

TAKE HEART

Are you a mover? Do you get regular exercise?

TAKE ACTION

Commit to walking at least thirty minutes three to five times this week.

JUST A TOUCH

God did extraordinary miracles through Paul, so that even hand-kerchiefs and aprons that had touched him were taken to the sick, and their illnesses were cured and the evil spirits left them.
—ACTS 19:11–12

G OD WAS (AND is) on the move. He was using Paul in a mighty way. It was so miraculous, even scarves and handkerchiefs that touched Paul's skin and were then taken to the sick brought healing and cast out demons. Incredible.

Now, remember, it's not the scarf or handkerchief that heals—it's God! Just a touch from God (sometimes through others) changes everything.

TAKE HEART

Was Paul special? Do you think this still happens?

TAKE ACTION

Are there things you have put your faith in over God? Food, medicine, man, vaccines, etc.? God can use anything or anyone, but remember, the healing comes from God himself.

A TRAGIC ACCIDENT REDEEMED

Because he intended to leave the next day, [Paul] kept on talking until midnight. Seated in a window was a young man named Eutychus, who was sinking into a deep sleep as Paul talked on and on. When he was sound asleep, he fell to the ground from the third story and was picked up dead. Paul went down, threw himself on the young man and put his arms around him. "Don't be alarmed," he said. "He's alive!" ...The people took the young man home alive and were greatly comforted.
—ACTS 20:7–12

SOMETIMES WHEN YOU read the Scriptures, they can almost make you laugh. This is one of those incredible, funny, miraculous stories. Paul was teaching and preaching late one night—and going "on and on." One of the guys fell asleep. That's the part that makes me laugh. I remember falling asleep as a little boy in the pews in church. However, the tragedy here is that this man then fell out of a three-story window and died. Paul went downstairs and lay on top of him, and he was raised from death to life! The people "were greatly comforted." What an incredible story!

TAKE HEART

This time a traumatic injury, not a disease, was healed. Have you considered praying for healing for this type of injury?

TAKE ACTION

I love Paul's boldness. You don't hear him say, "If it is Your will"; you just see action. Don't put conditions on your prayers.

Day 199
SNAKEBITES AND MORE HEALINGS

But Paul shook the snake off into the fire and suffered no ill effects. The people expected him to swell up or suddenly fall dead; but...seeing nothing unusual happen to him, they...said he was a god....Publius, the chief official of the island...welcomed us to his home....His father was sick in bed, suffering from fever and dysentery. Paul went in to see him and, after prayer, placed his hands on him and healed him. When this had happened, the rest of the sick on the island came and were cured.
—ACTS 28:5–9

WHEN THE SHIP Paul was on wrecked at Malta, the local islanders welcomed the people and built a fire for them. A venomous snake came out and bit Paul, and they thought he would die. But Paul just shook it off with no harm. Later Paul found out that the chief's father was sick. While visiting him, Paul prayed for him, and he was healed. As usual, once the people found out about this, all the sick "came and were cured."

I know we have read of so many healings and miracles, but each one is a critical, precious reminder of God's healing power. We often massively underappreciate it.

TAKE HEART

Do you take your eyesight, your heartbeat, and so on for granted? Think of all the miraculous things your body does every second.

TAKE ACTION

Say a prayer of thankfulness and gratitude for these things.

Day 200
PEACE AND JOY

*We boast in the hope of the glory of God. Not only so, but
we also glory in our sufferings, because we know that suffering produces perseverance; perseverance, character;
and character, hope. And hope does not put us to shame,
because God's love has been poured out into our hearts
through the Holy Spirit, who has been given to us.*
—ROMANS 5:2–5

WE ARE LIVING in a time of unprecedented stress, anxiety, fear, depression, addiction, and even suicide. The
numbers of people suffering right now are staggering. The
Scriptures are loaded with countless encouragements and perspectives that soothe the soul, mind, and spirit. Romans 5 is
one of them. It explains that even in the struggles, there is
purpose. We can rejoice in the pain and suffering because of
what we know it leads to. Praise the Lord!

The challenge in today's culture is that so many people
don't think they should have pain. So we self-medicate. These
are not the plans of God. He is our healer, protector, advocate,
and counselor. Take it to Him to find the purpose in the pain.

TAKE HEART

How do you respond to pain or trial? Do you look to man or
man-made solutions?

TAKE ACTION

Audit your life. Do you have a biblical perspective of suffering? If not, repent and pray for healing.

MORE SINNING = MORE GRACE?

*What shall we say, then? Shall we go on sinning
so that grace may increase? By no means! We are
those who have died to sin; how can we live in it any
longer? Or don't you know that all of us who were baptized into Christ Jesus were baptized into his death?*
—ROMANS 6:1–3

THERE IS OFTEN a mindset that can prevent God's gift of grace. It sounds something like this: "Well, since God has grace for me, it doesn't really matter what I do. He forgives me and we are good." Let me tell you this, and please hear this straight to your heart: God's grace and Jesus' death on the cross were not an endorsement of your sinful lifestyle. Without Jesus, the wages of sin are still death. God's grace is not a "get out of jail free" card. Only through Jesus can we be welcomed into God's kingdom. Paul basically says through new life in Christ, we are dead to sin. So any sin that is in our lives is a part of the old man and must be repented for; we cannot just be OK with it.

TAKE HEART

Do you think God is OK with sin in your life? Are you still praying for help to overcome that?

TAKE ACTION

List the sins that you can remember committing in the last twenty-four hours. Repent and pray.

Day 202
LIVE BY THE SPIRIT

*Those who live according to the flesh have their minds set on
what the flesh desires; but those who live in accordance with
the Spirit have their minds set on what the Spirit desires. The
mind governed by the flesh is death, but the mind governed by
the Spirit is life and peace....Those who are in the realm of the
flesh cannot please God. You, however, are...in the realm of
the Spirit, if indeed the Spirit of God lives in you. And if anyone
does not have the Spirit of Christ, they do not belong to Christ.*
—ROMANS 8:5–9

So MANY OF our problems, both physical and emotional,
occur because we operate in the flesh instead of in the
Holy Spirit. We find ourselves making short-sighted, fleshly
decisions that tend to lead us into sin. However, there is
another option—a better way, a higher road. When God lives
in us and we are baptized in the Holy Spirit, we can now
choose to live by the Spirit. It is an intentional choice—not
an easy one but one that makes all the difference. "There is a
way that appears to be right, but in the end it leads to death"
(Prov. 14:12).

TAKE HEART

Do you live by faith in the Spirit or fear in the flesh?

TAKE ACTION

Identify areas of known sin in your life. Ask the Lord to help
you see this from a spiritual perspective.

THE HOLY SPIRIT INTERCEDES

In the same way, the Spirit helps us in our weakness. We do not know what we ought to pray for, but the Spirit himself intercedes for us through wordless groans. And he who searches our hearts knows the mind of the Spirit, because the Spirit intercedes for God's people in accordance with the will of God. And we know that in all things God works for the good of those who love him, who have been called according to his purpose.
—ROMANS 8:26–28

THIS IS ONE of the most incredible scriptures. I really want you to consider what is being stated here. It tells us that the Holy Spirit himself intercedes and prays for us. *Mind blown.* When you are at a loss for words, at the end of your rope, and don't know what to pray, God the Holy Spirit intercedes and prays for you! If that doesn't provide immense peace and joy, I don't know what will. Amazing. If you struggle with anxiety, stress, or depression, this passage is for you. It's so rich with truth, power, and hope for believers, who have the Holy Spirit inside them.

TAKE HEART

Did you know this? How amazing it is that the Holy Spirit, Christ in you, prays for you.

TAKE ACTION

Reflect on all the times in your life that the Holy Spirit interceded for you and you didn't even know it. Give thanks.

BUT THAT'S NOT FAIR

*What then shall we say? Is God unjust? Not at all! For he
says to Moses, "I will have mercy on whom I have mercy,
and I will have compassion on whom I have compassion."*
—ROMANS 9:14–15

OH HOW WE like to get mad at God at times. We don't
like when someone else gets mercy or is healed, forgiven,
or blessed. We often get bitter and depressed and say, "What
about me, God?" The root of this thought is pride. We think
more of ourselves than we ought to, and out of that sin of
pride, we tend to take matters into our own hands. We don't
like how God is doing it, but who are we to question His ways,
even when we don't like them? And if we are honest, we are
mostly seeking our own comfort and selfish desires. *Lord, we
need You! Help us be free from ourselves.*

TAKE HEART

Be honest with yourself. How do you feel when God seems to
be moving in a mighty way in someone else's life, especially
if it's someone you don't like? What if others get healed in an
area where you need one? Or they get married and you are
feeling lonely? Just be honest: How do you feel?

TAKE ACTION

Take these feelings to God. Let Him give you a new and better
perspective—a godly one. *Lord, let us see the way You see.*

Day 205
MIC DROP!

Therefore, I urge you, brothers and sisters, in view of God's mercy, to offer your bodies as a living sacrifice, holy and pleasing to God—this is your true and proper worship.
—ROMANS 12:1

THIS IS AN amazing passage of Scripture that in some ways sums up the prayer I have for this book and for you: that we offer our bodies as living sacrifices, "holy and pleasing to God," which is a spiritual act of worship.

I think this is the perfect perspective we need for our temporary physical bodies. It removes the vanity and pride. Caring for yourself should not be self-worship; it's worship to God. In a time where everything is about self, it is critical that we see self-care through God's eyes, offering our bodies as living sacrifices.

TAKE HEART

Is this how you view your body? Does this change your perspective on wellness and health?

TAKE ACTION

List all the ways you can worship through caring for your body, such as working out for Jesus, eating well for Jesus, resting for Jesus, etc.

Day 206
RENEW YOUR MIND

Do not conform to the pattern of this world, but be transformed by the renewing of your mind. Then you will be able to test and approve what God's will is—his good, pleasing and perfect will.
—ROMANS 12:2

WHAT A TIMELY scripture. An amazing aspect of scriptural truth is how it remains relevant and timeless. In today's confusing culture, it is absolutely essential that we renew our minds daily so we test and approve God's will.

How do we do that? What does it take to renew our minds? Well, let's start with what it doesn't: social media, mainstream media, gossip. Instead, these are some things we know will help: reading, meditating on, and listening to the Word of God; praying; worshipping; journaling; and so on. If you are currently spending a lot of time in the world, it is affecting you negatively—period. Make moves to get outside the ways of the world.

TAKE HEART

Are you spending too much time in the world, on social media, on Netflix, etc.?

TAKE ACTION

Log off. Get off social media for thirty days. Put the TV in the closet. Cancel Netflix. You won't regret it.

MANY PARTS, ONE BODY

So we, being many, are one body in Christ,
and all are parts of one another.
—ROMANS 12:5, MEV

ILOVE LEARNING INTERESTING, amazing facts about the human body. It reminds me of all the metaphors in Scripture related to the body. Just as each organ has a particular function, we all play different but important roles in the body of Christ.

God does so much for us and our bodies on a daily basis that we simply don't realize it or we take it for granted. The saliva He created in our mouths to begin proper digestion is one of them. Incredible! *Thank You, Jesus, for these amazing bodies.*

TAKE HEART

When is the last time you thanked God for your spit? How many things does God do every day in the body He gave you that you don't even think about or thank Him for?

TAKE ACTION

Thank God for your saliva. As you eat or swallow, take notice how phenomenal these simple acts are. Blinking, breathing, bathroom breaks, walking—they're all *amazing!*

Day 208

SOME PRACTICAL TEACHING

Love must be sincere. Hate what is evil; cling to what
is good. Be devoted to one another in love....Do not
be overcome by evil, but overcome evil with good.
—ROMANS 12:9–10, 21

SOMETIMES THE BIBLE requires deep, thoughtful prayer and meditation and contains mysteries. And other times it is pretty straightforward. This is one of those times.

"Hate what is evil; cling to what is good." That's a pretty good start. In today's contrary world, this can actually seem confusing as the world attempts to redefine good and evil. I appreciate the following quote: "Truth sounds like hate to those who hate the truth."[1] So it is important that we have a biblical understanding of what is good and evil.

The devil likes to confuse. God is good. Jesus is good. The devil is evil. He came to steal, kill, and destroy. If you want to know good, know God. Study His Word and His ways. There is no other way. It is worth it. Know God; know good.

TAKE HEART

Do you struggle living this out in these times when some see biblical Christianity as hate speech?

TAKE ACTION

Don't let culture define good and evil. How do you define it?

208   *DESIGNED TO HEAL*

TRIGGER WARNING FOR GERMAPHOBES

Now may the God of perseverance and encouragement grant you to live in harmony with one another in accordance with Christ Jesus.
—ROMANS 15:5, MEV

YOU HAVE TRILLIONS of viruses and bacteria in you right now! And they are *good* for you![1] The world has created so much fear around germs and viruses. As I've heard people say, "If germs killed us, we would all be dead."[2]

Of course, there are germs and viruses everywhere, and there always will be. The most important thing to remember and focus on is not the germ but the *host* or the *soil*. As long as we are healthy, our bodies live in harmony with germs.

TAKE HEART

What do you think about the fact that you have trillions of germs in and on you all the time? Gross? Cool? Amazing? Scary?

TAKE ACTION

Take some time to reconsider your fear of all things germ-related. Consider areas you have been misled to fear germs. God made germs too.

MAN'S WISDOM?

*For the foolishness of God is wiser than human wisdom, and
the weakness of God is stronger than human strength.*
—1 CORINTHIANS 1:25

IT'S EASY TO think that we have it all figured out. We look
at smartphones and space rockets and pat ourselves on the
back like we humans are so smart. It's kind of like we say to
God, "Thank You for everything, but we will take it from
here." Oh the hubris.

Scripture says God's foolishness is wiser than man's wisdom.
Truth. Some have estimated that we know less than 1 percent
about the human body, but look how cocky and arrogant we
are about health and manipulating God's design with pills,
potions, drugs, and surgery. In all of human history, we have
never created a single living cell, yet God does it in your body
daily without you even thinking about it. It would serve us and
God well if we operated with the perspective that He is God
and we are not.

TAKE HEART

Do you find yourself thinking more about you than God? We
make idols of people like Elon Musk and Mark Zuckerberg,
but do we even talk about who created it all?

TAKE ACTION

Give God the glory. He is the creator and sustainer of all
things. Look at God's creation, and be in awe.

Day 211
KEEP IT SIMPLE

*But God has chosen the foolish things of the world to
confound the wise. God has chosen the weak things of
the world to confound the things which are mighty.*
—1 CORINTHIANS 1:27, MEV

SOMETIMES WE JUST need to keep it simple. Jesus loves
me; this I know. His grace is sufficient. It is by faith we
are saved. And we need to eat less CRAP: carbonated drinks,
refined sugar, artificial sweeteners, and processed food. Sometimes we can overwhelm ourselves and complicate the process,
and we end up giving up before we even start.

TAKE HEART

Remember, Jesus paid a high price for our lives and bodies
(1 Cor. 6:20). We are created in His likeness and image. Our
bodies are temples of the Holy Spirit. We are commanded to
care for the bodies God gave us. Are you doing that?

TAKE ACTION

For one week, avoid CRAP. How do you think you will feel?

EYES TO SEE

But as it is written, "Eye has not seen, nor ear heard,
nor has it entered into the heart of man the things
which God has prepared for those who love Him."
—1 CORINTHIANS 2:9, MEV

YOU BLINK ABOUT 28,800 times a day. *Give us eyes to see, Lord!* We take so many parts of the body (and the body of Christ) for granted. The simple involuntary, automatic action of blinking literally allows us to see by keeping our eyes moist and healthy! The design of the eye is so profound and complex that there is much we still don't understand about it. Imagine being blind. Imagine being blind to Jesus! Open your eyes to the fullness of Jesus and what He has for you.

TAKE HEART

The human eye can differentiate about ten million different colors.[1] Are you seeing all the things God wants you to see?

TAKE ACTION

We are called to view people according to their hearts or spirits, not their outer appearance. Is there anyone or anything you need to see differently?

Day 213
WISDOM FROM THE SPIRIT

No one knows the thoughts of God except the Spirit of
God. What we have received is...the Spirit who is from
God, so that we may understand what God has freely
given us. This is what we speak...explaining spiritual reali-
ties with Spirit-taught words. The person without the Spirit
does not accept the things that come from the Spirit of God
but considers them foolishness, and cannot understand
them because they are discerned only through the Spirit.
—1 CORINTHIANS 2:11–14

THANK GOD HE sent His Spirit to us after Christ's death
and resurrection. The fact that He resides inside us, Christ
in us, is a game changer. This scripture from Paul reminds us
of the difference that operating from the Spirit makes. People
who do not have the Spirit will not understand. It will actually
look like foolishness. But the Spirit of God within us knows
God's nature. The wisdom of God—the wisdom of the Holy
Spirit—is within us. We must surrender and follow the Spirit,
not the flesh. Yes, it is the road less traveled. Yes, many will
not understand. But it is the way of wisdom and truth.

TAKE HEART

Are you led more by the Spirit or by the flesh? Have you experienced wisdom that could come only from God?

TAKE ACTION

Resist battling worldly ideas with other worldly ideas. Be
intentional about seeking the Spirit's wisdom, not man's.

DESIGNED TO HEAL

Day 214
FEED YOUR BRAIN!

For, "Who has known the mind of the Lord so as to instruct him?" But we have the mind of Christ.
—1 CORINTHIANS 2:16

THE RESEARCH OF Roger W. Sperry, a Nobel Prize recipient, showed that "90% of the stimulation and nutrition to the brain is generated by the movement of the spine."[1] This is an amazing way to look at movement and exercise! Think of exercise as food for the brain. Numerous studies show one of the most important things we can do to guard against Alzheimer's is to stay active. You are designed to move—a lot. Don't take for granted the body God gave you. Use it.

TAKE HEART

Have you ever thought about exercise as food for your brain? Are you feeding your brain well?

TAKE ACTION

If you have concerns about mental health or neurodegenerative disease, it is really important that you move your body. Find a friend or family member to be active with. Get a dog to take on walks. Just do something. You will never regret it.

Day 215

THE TEMPLE OF THE HOLY SPIRIT, PART 1

*What? Do you not know that your body is the temple
of the Holy Spirit, who is in you, whom you have
received from God, and that you are not your own?*
—1 CORINTHIANS 6:19, MEV

EACH CAN OF soda has about ten to thirteen teaspoons of sugar in it. That much sugar can seriously affect your immune system. Imagine if you are living on that much sugar several times a day! Research has shown that consuming 75 grams of sugar (which is less than two cans of soda) can significantly reduce immune system function for up to five hours![1] It is no surprise we get sick.

TAKE HEART

Are you addicted to sugar? Have you ever considered what your food choices may be doing to your health?

TAKE ACTION

Try a sugar fast or sugar detox. You may not feel great for a few days, but it is worth it. *You* are worth it. Do it for yourself or your family. Or do it as a form of worship to Jesus.

THE TEMPLE OF THE HOLY SPIRIT, PART 2

What? Do you not know that your body is the temple of the Holy Spirit, who is in you, whom you have received from God, and that you are not your own?
—1 CORINTHIANS 6:19, MEV

REMEMBER THE OLD saying "You are what you eat"? We used to laugh about that as kids, but the truth is, it is pretty accurate. Our bodies take the nutrients from the food we eat and repair, rebuild, and regenerate our bodies. If you are living on Twinkies, whiskey, and potato chips, you are not rebuilding a strong body. The best body-rebuilding materials are foods made by God, such as fruits, vegetables, and nuts.

TAKE HEART

If you took all the food you ate in the last week and put it in a big bowl, would this be good fuel and materials for your body to repair and rebuild from?

TAKE ACTION

Add water and real, God-created food to your day and see how you feel.

THE TEMPLE OF THE HOLY SPIRIT, PART 3

What? Do you not know that your body is the temple of the Holy Spirit, who is in you, whom you have received from God, and that you are not your own? You were bought with a price. Therefore glorify God in your body and in your spirit, which are God's.
—1 CORINTHIANS 6:19–20, MEV

PROBABLY ONE OF the most common objections to eating healthy is that it is too high-priced. No doubt healthy food can be a bit more expensive; however, you are worth it! In working with patients for over twenty years, I have found that most people can find a way to eat healthy on a budget. Often we just need to get rid of the junk we have been eating.

TAKE HEART

We are what we eat. Are you eating dirty or clean? Our moods, hormones, energy, health, and so much more can easily be affected by what we eat.

TAKE ACTION

Learn to be savvy at the store. What are some toxic foods you need to take out of your diet? What are some clean ones you can add?

IS FOOD AN IDOL TO YOU?

*There is but one God, the Father, from whom all things came
and for whom we live; and there is but one Lord, Jesus
Christ, through whom all things came and through whom
we live....Some people are still so accustomed to idols that
when they eat sacrificial food they think of it as having been
sacrificed to a god, and since their conscience is weak, it
is defiled. But food does not bring us near to God; we
are no worse if we do not eat, and no better if we do.*
—1 CORINTHIANS 8:6–8

IN THIS INTERESTING but somewhat confusing passage, Paul
discusses food that has been sacrificed to idols and when
it is appropriate to eat certain types of food. He asks us to be
considerate of our fellow believers and others who may see us.

Food has become such an idol for both believers and non-
believers. We often make so much fuss about food. Many
scriptures, especially in the New Testament, can help set us
free from this idol, which can cause guilt, shame, gluttony,
fear, disease, etc. How is your relationship with food? How
big of a role does it play in your life?

TAKE HEART

God gave us food. It is good. But have you given it more
authority than it deserves?

TAKE ACTION

Reflect on how you feel about food and God. Pray about it. Do
you have an unhealthy relationship with food?

FLEE EVIL

Therefore, my dear friends, flee from idolatry.
—1 CORINTHIANS 10:14

IT IS CRITICAL to remember that our skin absorbs whatever is applied to it. These chemicals then circulate through the entire body and can have all sorts of different effects. Many of us have made idols of our looks and bodies, but at what cost? It is amazing to look back just a few years and see how things change. Chemicals and drugs we thought were "safe" or "good for us" have now been shown to be dangerous or even deadly.

As believers, we need to be discerning about what we take into our minds and hearts. There are many things the world tells us are good but are actually deadly. As the old saying goes, "Hindsight is twenty-twenty."

TAKE HEART

The flesh is weak; modern marketers and purveyors of media propaganda know this. It is critical we guard our hearts against the agendas of this world.

TAKE ACTION

What things you are doing today might prove to be a problem in the future? Address these now.

Day 220
GIVE GOD THE GLORY

*Whether you eat or drink or whatever you do, do it all for the
glory of God. Do not cause anyone to stumble...even as I try
to please everyone in every way. For I am not seeking my
own good but the good of many, so that they may be saved.*
—1 Corinthians 10:31–33

HERE AGAIN WE see some good instructions about how we
are to engage with food and drink and others. It seems
Paul is exposing what still happens today. We make food all
about us—what we want, what we are in the mood for, etc. But
Paul cuts right through it all by reminding us to do it all for
the glory of God.

This kingdom-minded perspective is a whole different level.
It challenges us to reflect on food and see it from a spiritual
perspective. For example, what if you were with some great
friends and they brought some food you wouldn't normally
eat? Do you think it would be for the glory of God to simply
be thankful and enjoy the fellowship? Give thanks for the
food God has provided. Give thanks for those who have prepared it and those you eat it with. Don't make food a bigger
deal than it is.

TAKE HEART

Do you eat for the glory of God?

TAKE ACTION

Say grace before every meal. Thank God for the food.

FOOD AS A STRONGHOLD?

For he who eats and drinks unworthily, eats and drinks dam-
nation to himself, not discerning the Lord's body. For this
reason many are weak and unhealthy among you, and many
die. If we would judge ourselves, we would not be judged.
—1 CORINTHIANS 11:29–31, MEV

THE UNITED STATES is leading the way in one area of health metrics: we have one of the highest rates of obesity on earth.[1] We must remember gluttony is a sin. We have idolized food so much in the last several years, people identify as "foodies" and spend time taking pictures of food and planning their next meals. All this excessive attention to food, particularly the idolizing of food, has not made us healthier. And all the predictions say it will only get worse. We have more obese kids now than ever before. And the current medical answer is to start medicating these kids.

TAKE HEART

God did not create us to be sick, overweight, and literally eating ourselves into disease and suffering. What do you think about these statistics? What do you think God thinks? Why does the church not address these issues very often?

TAKE ACTION

Is food an idol in your life? Eat to live; don't live to eat. Yes, God created food for us, but not so we could be controlled by it. He made it to sustain us so we can do the things He has called us to do.

Day 222
GIFTS OF THE SPIRIT

There are different kinds of gifts, but the same Spirit distributes them....Now to each one the manifestation of the Spirit is given for the common good. To one there is given through the Spirit a message of wisdom, to another a message of knowledge...to another faith...to another gifts of healing...to another miraculous powers, to another prophecy, to another distinguishing between spirits, to another speaking in different kinds of tongues, and to still another the interpretation of tongues. All these are the work of one and the same Spirit, and he distributes them to each one, just as he determines.
—1 CORINTHIANS 12:4–11

DISCUSSIONS ABOUT THE gifts of the Spirit can get "spirited" at times because of different perspectives. But I think we can all agree we are to use any spiritual gift we receive to serve others and glorify God. So many times we turn God's gifts into selfish tools instead of blessings to others. All good gifts are from the Lord. We need to remain humble and mindful of that. The gifts are not so we can make more of ourselves but so we can make more of Him and serve others.

TAKE HEART

What gifts has God given you? How are you using them to bless and edify others?

TAKE ACTION

Have you thanked God for His gifts? Have you asked Him to show you how to use them to serve others?

Day 223
ALL TOGETHER NOW

The body is not one part, but many. If the foot says, "Because I am not the hand, I am not of the body," is it therefore not of the body? And if the ear says, "Because I am not the eye, I am not of the body," is it therefore not of the body? If the whole body were an eye, where would the hearing be? If the whole body were hearing, where would the sense of smell be? But now God has established the parts, every one of them, in the body as it has pleased Him. If they were all one part, where would the body be?
—1 CORINTHIANS 12:14–19, MEV

A POSTER OF THE autonomic nervous system really changed how I saw the body God created for me. (See appendix.) It showed me how the nerves connect to all my organs and enter my spine and helped me see the incredible relationship among all these.

Do you know how healthy your spine is? Have you ever had it examined or x-rayed? It just may be the ticket to getting to the root of some of your health concerns.

TAKE HEART

The more you learn about how God created your body, the more awe and reverence you will have for it.

TAKE ACTION

Pick one area of the body to learn about. Google some amazing facts about it. And remember, some say we know less than 1 percent about how the human body works.

BODY OF CHRIST

*The eye cannot say to the hand, "I don't need you!"...On
the contrary, those parts of the body that seem to be
weaker are indispensable, and the parts that we think are
less honorable we treat with special honor....But God has
put the body together...so that there should be no divi-
sion in the body, but that its parts should have equal concern for each other. If one part suffers, every part suffers
with it; if one part is honored, every part rejoices with it.*
—1 CORINTHIANS 12:21–26

IN THE BODY of Christ, we all play different roles. One is
an eye, another a hand; some are parts we see; others are
hidden. But they are all equal and important. Much stress
can come when God made you an "ear" but you want to be a
"hand." Some people live their whole lives wanting to be something or someone other than who God made them to be. Few
things are worse than missing out on the specific, special role
God has uniquely created for you.

Don't fall into the deadly trap of comparison. Operate in
the gifts and calling God has for you. You matter. You have a
specific, vital role in the body of Christ.

TAKE HEART

Have you talked to God about your part in the body of Christ?

TAKE ACTION

Reflect on times you have been jealous or envious. How did
that work out?

Day 225
LOVE IS...

Love is patient, love is kind. It does not envy, it does not boast, it is not proud. It does not dishonor others, it is not self-seeking, it is not easily angered, it keeps no record of wrongs. Love does not delight in evil but rejoices with the truth. It always protects, always trusts, always hopes, always perseveres.
—1 CORINTHIANS 13:4–7

YOU HAVE PROBABLY heard this "love" passage read at weddings. It is very powerful to use as a reflection to see how well we are loving. God is love. We are called to be Christlike and love each other. So what does it say here about love? And how we are doing?

Love (God) is patient; are you? Love (God) is kind; are you? Love (God) does not envy; do you? Love (God) does not boast; do you? Love (God) is not proud; are you? Love (God) is not rude; are you? Love (God) is not self-seeking; are you? Love (God) is not easily annoyed; are you? Love (God) keeps no record of wrongs; do you? Love (God) rejoices in truth; do you? Love (God) always protects, always trusts, always hopes, always perseveres; do you?

TAKE HEART

How did you do?

TAKE ACTION

Pick one or two areas to focus on to improve.

Day 226
BE A LIVER

For as in Adam all die, so in Christ all will be made alive.
—1 CORINTHIANS 15:22

MY FAVORITE ORGAN name is the liver. We all want to be alive. We all want to be livers! Your liver is one of the most amazing organisms. It makes cholesterol, hormones, and vitamin D. This is simply a reminder of the incredible intricacies of your body. You can actually remove 75 percent of your liver and it will *regrow* in six to eight weeks! Isn't God amazing?

TAKE HEART

When is the last time, if ever, you considered your liver and all the things it does without you knowing or thinking about it?

TAKE ACTION

Give God thanks for your liver! Be a *liver* not a *dier*.

THE GOD OF ALL COMFORT

Praise be to...the Father of compassion and the God of all comfort, who comforts us in all our troubles, so that we can comfort those in any trouble....For just as we share abundantly in the sufferings of Christ, so also our comfort abounds through Christ. If we are distressed, it is for your comfort and salvation; if we are comforted, it is for your comfort, which produces in you patient endurance....And our hope for you is firm, because we know that just as you share in our sufferings, so also you share in our comfort.
—2 Corinthians 1:3–7

As a doctor I meet so many people struggling with stress, anxiety, and depression. And recent times have brought more stress for people. Fear, worry, and stress can make us go to the world and make bad decisions—we lose faith and fall away; we feel God isn't there; we feel lost. There will always be things to worry and stress about, things of real concern. But God has something to say about that. These scriptures are so powerful. If you are in a place where you need His comfort and peace, this passage, this truth, is for you. Read it over and over.

Take Heart

Where do you go when you are stressed out? What does God's Word say?

Take Action

Find two or three scriptures that talk about God's promises and comfort. If you are struggling, read and memorize these verses.

BLINDED BY THE LIGHT

The god of this age has blinded the minds of unbelievers,
so that they cannot see the light of the gospel that dis-
plays the glory of Christ, who is the image of God.
—2 CORINTHIANS 4:4

WE ARE COMMANDED to let our light shine; however, sometimes through our lifestyle or the trials of life, the light is diminished. There is research that shows chiropractic adjustments help us to function and live more resilient lives.

Studies have looked at the brain's activity before and after chiropractic adjustments. The results are amazing. The brain and nerve system are better able to handle stress *after* an adjustment. I have delivered about 1.5 million adjustments in my life and have heard countless stories of how much better and more relaxed people feel after being adjusted.

TAKE HEART

Even your brain is designed to heal through what is called neuroplasticity. Your brain is constantly adapting and learning. The Scriptures talk often about renewing our minds. God wouldn't tell us to do that if it wasn't possible. You can rewire the brain by changing the way you think.

TAKE ACTION

Get a chiropractic adjustment. There are many different styles and techniques, but they all help balance the nerve system.

LIVING BY FAITH, NOT BY SIGHT

We live by faith, not by sight.
—2 CORINTHIANS 5:7

SEVEN WORDS. THIS scripture seems like such a simple concept. It even makes a nice inspirational quote or T-shirt.
But when we actually have to put faith in action, when we
have to step out, when we have to get real with our faith, it
gets scary.

I think this is what holds so many of us back. We live by
sight, not by faith. But let me challenge that in a few practical ways. Last night when you went to sleep, your heart
kept beating. How? Do you have faith that it will continue?
If you're married, you took that step in faith that you will be
together forever. Maybe you decided to have kids, even with
all the risks and concerns and responsibility. You took a job;
you drive a car.

Every day of our lives is a new adventure, and we don't
know what will come our way. We live by faith, whether we
like it or believe it. The question then becomes, What do we
have faith in, and how much faith do we have?

TAKE HEART

Would you consider yourself a faith-filled person?

TAKE ACTION

Reflect on areas you need more faith. Ask God.

A NEW CREATION

*Therefore, if anyone is in Christ, the new creation
has come: The old has gone, the new is here! All this
is from God, who reconciled us to himself through
Christ and gave us the ministry of reconciliation.*
—2 CORINTHIANS 5:17–18

IT IS FASCINATING how much the Scriptures talk about perspective, mind, and attitude. If ever there was a book discussing mental health and wellness, the Bible sure is an amazing one. But this passage is one that we really need to meditate on and think about the implications. If you are "in Christ," the Holy Spirit lives in you, and you are new. The old nature is gone. You are born again, and all of that is from God. This is not a metaphor or hyperbole. This is a literal statement. You are a new person. Now, it's possible that you may not feel new. That's where sanctification comes in. That's where we need to mature in our relationships with the Lord. But a miracle has happened. You are a new creation. The old is gone.

TAKE HEART

Do you believe this? Why or why not?

TAKE ACTION

If you are a new person, act like it. Think about being married—time to grow up and take responsibility. Do your part. God has.

AND YOU THINK YOU HAVE HAD IT ROUGH

As servants of God we commend ourselves...in great endurance; in troubles, hardships and distresses; in beatings, imprisonments and riots; in hard work, sleepless nights and hunger... in the Holy Spirit and in sincere love...genuine, yet regarded as impostors; known, yet regarded as unknown...beaten, and yet not killed; sorrowful, yet always rejoicing; poor, yet making many rich; having nothing, and yet possessing everything. We have spoken freely...and opened wide our hearts to you....As a fair exchange...open wide your hearts also.
—2 CORINTHIANS 6:3–13

REMEMBER PAUL? HE had a dramatic encounter with Jesus. He went from murdering and imprisoning Christians to writing much of the New Testament. Paul also went through persecution—being stoned, shipwrecked, beaten, imprisoned, and more. Yet even with all that, he had a wide-open heart.

This passage should humble and amaze us at the same time. Paul is calling us out, from a place of love. He's telling us to have open hearts. And Paul has the authority to speak this into us because he lived it without becoming hardened.

TAKE HEART

Is your heart is open, or do you need a new perspective?

TAKE ACTION

Reflect on areas you may have developed a closed, hard heart. Ask God to soften and rescue you from that.

Day 232

BE CAREFUL WHOM YOU YOKE WITH

Do not be yoked together with unbelievers. For what do righteousness and wickedness have in common? Or what fellowship can light have with darkness?...Or what does a believer have in common with an unbeliever? What agreement is there between the temple of God and idols? For we are the temple of the living God. As God has said: "I will live with them and walk among them...." Therefore, "Come out from them and be separate, says the Lord."
—2 CORINTHIANS 6:14–17

I THINK 2 CORINTHIANS needs to be rereleased today to help pull so many believers out of their funk. We need a fresh perspective on how to engage with a messy, sinful, dark world. Paul does not beat around the bush. If you or someone you know struggles in this area, here is some kingdom advice. Don't mess with darkness. Don't dabble with sin. Don't justify living with the devil. Seek God. Yes, there is a time to evangelize, but we don't have anything in common with wickedness. Remember, we are new creations in Christ. Take responsibility for the things you surround yourself with.

TAKE HEART

When you look at your life and relationships, are you spending your time on righteous things? What would Jesus say to you?

TAKE ACTION

What or whom do you need to unyoke from? Take a step toward that today.

232   *DESIGNED TO HEAL*

PURIFY

*Therefore, since we have these promises, dear friends, let
us purify ourselves from everything that contaminates body
and spirit, perfecting holiness out of reverence for God.*
—2 CORINTHIANS 7:1

T HIS IS A big verse. I am going to take it point by point:

- "Since we have these promises"—you have promises from God. You can take them to the bank.
  Trust Him, even if it's hard. He's a promise keeper.

- "Let us purify ourselves from everything that contaminates body and spirit"—we need to clean
  ourselves, both physically and spiritually, of the
  junk we feed our bodies and minds.

- "Perfecting holiness out of reverence for God"—
  this is how we worship and glorify God. If we
  honor and glorify God, He empowers us to be
  holy.

TAKE HEART

What do you think when you read this? Does it seem too
hard? Too good to be true?

TAKE ACTION

Being holy is a way to glorify God. We are called to be holy.
We can do that only with Jesus. Is there an area in which you
need to come into obedience? Ask the Lord to empower you
to make the needed changes.

GODLY SORROW

I am happy...because your sorrow led you to repentance....
Godly sorrow brings repentance that leads to salvation and
leaves no regret, but worldly sorrow brings death. See what
this godly sorrow has produced in you: what earnestness, what
eagerness to clear yourselves, what indignation, what alarm,
what longing, what concern, what readiness to see justice done.
—2 CORINTHIANS 7:9–11

SOMETIMES WE NEED to be called out on our stuff. We need a bold, godly friend to help us see that what we are doing is not OK in God's eyes. The "godly sorrow" this produces leads to real, authentic repentance, which leads to salvation and rescue from God. It gives us His heart and perspective.

Worldly sorrow brings death, but godly sorrow brings life. Godly sorrow changes us deeply. It makes us more like God. So much of the guilt, shame, and "not good enough" feelings we experience are not godly sorrow. They're a fallen world trying to entice us into sin. Let us not fall for the trap but celebrate when we experience godly sorrow, holy discontent.

TAKE HEART

Have you ever experienced godly sorrow? Felt convicted by the Holy Spirit? Did it change you?

TAKE ACTION

Reflect on times you have felt guilty or "bad." Where did those feelings come from: God or the world? Be intentional about being bothered by sins against God.

DO YOU HAVE A GENEROUS HEART?

We want you to know about the grace that God has given the Macedonian churches. In the midst of a very severe trial, their overflowing joy and their extreme poverty welled up in rich generosity. For I testify that they gave as much as they were able, and even beyond their ability....And they exceeded our expectations: They gave themselves first of all to the Lord, and then by the will of God also to us....But since you excel in everything...see that you also excel in this grace of giving.
—2 CORINTHIANS 8:1–7

D O YOU CONSIDER yourself generous? What is the standard you use to measure that? Studies about giving have shown that an average of 5 percent of churchgoers tithe and they give about 2.5 percent of their income.[1] Hmm. Well, this passage tells us an amazing story about generosity. It starts with "the grace that God has given." The only way we will be generous like our perfect Father in heaven is if He gives us the grace. Another incredible part of the story is that the believers were in extreme poverty but "welled up in rich generosity." Wow, what an astonishing picture of God's grace and Spirit-led generosity. Let us be a people who joyfully give, even in our poverty.

TAKE HEART

If this is the standard, are you a generous, joyful giver?

TAKE ACTION

Pray that a spirit of generosity would well up in your spirit right now. Now take action—go give something to someone!

Day 236
REAP WHAT YOU SOW

*Whoever sows sparingly will also reap sparingly, and whoever
sows generously will also reap generously. Each of you should
give what you have decided in your heart to give, not reluctantly
or under compulsion, for God loves a cheerful giver. And God
is able to bless you abundantly, so that in all things at all times,
having all that you need, you will abound in every good work.*
—2 CORINTHIANS 9:6–8

THE BIBLE HAS deep practical wisdom. These words about
generosity are no different. God is clear: you get what you
give. Give little; receive little. I grew up in the Midwest "farm
country." If you desire a big harvest, you'd better plant a lot of
seeds in the spring. Paul gives us some additional godly suggestions: (1) Give God what you have decided in your heart,
and (2) know God will give you grace so that in all things, at
all times, you have all that you need.

You cannot outgive God. Remember, this is the God who
made everything out of nothing. He makes your heart beat;
He hung the stars. He is the Alpha and the Omega. He is
worthy of our trust and generosity. Never forget—it's His
grace that allows us to be generous.

TAKE HEART

Do you want to be generous? What holds you back?

TAKE ACTION

Reread God's promises related to generosity. If you want to
reap a lot, be generous.

TAKE EVERY THOUGHT CAPTIVE

For though we live in the world, we do not wage war as the world does. The weapons we fight with are not the weapons of the world. On the contrary, they have divine power to demolish strongholds. We demolish arguments and every pretension that sets itself up against the knowledge of God, and we take captive every thought to make it obedient to Christ.
—2 CORINTHIANS 10:3–5

IF EVER THERE was a primary issue I see crippling so many believers today, it is this one. We passively allow so many thoughts and so much information into our eyes, ears, minds, hearts, and souls. It is captivating areas of our hearts, and we are suffering because of it.

Paul lays it out clearly. Take every thought captive to obey Christ. Another way to say it is to be very careful what you think about and allow into your spirit. Garbage in; garbage out. We are not immune to things we see, hear, and feel. We need to be careful. If you are or have been exposed to impure things, take the thought captive so it does not take root.

TAKE HEART

Are you careful about what you expose your mind, eyes, and heart to? How about your kids?

TAKE ACTION

Be on guard. Do an audit of shows you watch, books you read, people in your life, and music you listen to. What would Jesus think?

Day 238

HIS GRACE IS SUFFICIENT

To keep me from becoming conceited, I was given a thorn in my flesh, a messenger of Satan, to torment me. Three times I pleaded with the Lord to take it away from me. But he said to me, "My grace is sufficient for you, for my power is made perfect in weakness." Therefore I will boast all the more gladly about my weaknesses, so that Christ's power may rest on me.
—2 CORINTHIANS 12:7–9

ITHINK WE ALL agree Paul was an amazingly committed follower of Jesus and the Lord was gracious to him. With that understanding it is fascinating to think that out of God's goodness, to keep Paul from becoming conceited, God allowed a "thorn" from Satan to harass him. When Paul begged the Lord to remove it, He refused, saying His grace was sufficient!

Just think through this. The Lord allowed a messenger of Satan to go after the great apostle Paul to keep him from becoming too proud! Wow. It is so easy to get mad at God when He allows bad things to happen. Even the greatest, godliest people experience bad things. God's reassurance for when this happens is "My grace is sufficient."

TAKE HEART

Do you get angry at God for things? Have you been angry when things seem unfair?

TAKE ACTION

Talk to God about these things, and ask Him what He is trying to show you.

ARE YOU SEEKING APPROVAL OF MAN OR GOD?

Am I now trying to win the approval of human beings, or of
God? Or am I trying to please people? If I were still trying
to please people, I would not be a servant of Christ.
—GALATIANS 1:10

SO MUCH OF today's stress and strife is caused by seeking favor from man. This causes so much perversion and sin in our lives. We chase the wind. Instead of being servants of Christ, we seek pleasure and man's approval. These next few thoughts might sting a little: we try to please our kids; we try to please our spouses; we try to please our bosses; we try to please our parents.

We often do some crazy things to please people and not even give a second thought to God. Ouch. We are called to serve God first. We must be very careful to not make our jobs, kids, spouses, money, friends, and health idols in our lives. You cannot chase two rabbits at once. Anything—even a "good" thing—can be an idol.

TAKE HEART

Are you serving God or man?

TAKE ACTION

Reflect on your day. Do you have some idols? What are you going to do? Serve God or serve man?

Day 240

FOURTEEN YEARS

*Then after fourteen years, I went up again to Jerusalem....I
went in response to a revelation and, meeting privately with
those esteemed as leaders, I presented to them the gospel
that I preach among the Gentiles. I wanted to be sure I was
not running and had not been running my race in vain.*
—GALATIANS 2:1–2

IT IS OFTEN said that we live in a quick-fix society. We want
everything yesterday. The Bible is certainly full of many
instantaneous miracles. But it is also full of examples of
patience, time, and process. David was anointed as king, but
it was fifteen to twenty years before he took the throne.

We live in time of immediacy, and we desire quick fixes. It
is important to remember that many of the faithful leaders in
Scripture spent years to decades waiting, seeking, and being
sanctified until the time was right. The Lord is often working
on many areas of our hearts to heal, restore, and redeem. He
is a God of miracles and process. What do you think God was
doing in Paul for those fourteen years?

TAKE HEART

How do you respond when God requires process? What can
we learn from Paul?

TAKE ACTION

Are there experiences you have stopped pursuing because it
was taking too long? Rethink this. God's timing is different
from ours.

Day 241
"I NO LONGER LIVE"

I have been crucified with Christ and I no longer live, but
Christ lives in me. The life I now live in the body, I live by
faith in the Son of God, who loved me and gave himself for
me. I do not set aside the grace of God, for if righteousness
could be gained through the law, Christ died for nothing!
—GALATIANS 2:20–21

THIS IS A mind-blowing, life-changing, perspective-shifting, soul-healing scripture. Honestly, if you are struggling with your purpose, journey, life…this scripture is an anchor. I am going to work backward through it.

"The Son of God (Jesus), who loved me and gave himself for me." Wow. He loved you first, while you were at your worst, and gave Himself for you! If you ever doubt your worth, read this scripture relentlessly. "The life I now live in the body, I live by faith in the Son of God." So let's follow this: Because of His love for you, Jesus gave Himself for you, and because of that great exchange, you can now live by faith in Him! "I have been crucified with Christ and I no longer live, but Christ lives in me." Because of what Christ did for us, we surrender our lives to Him.

TAKE HEART

How does this scripture make you feel?

TAKE ACTION

Write in a journal about how this affects and impacts you.

Day 242
WHO BEWITCHED YOU?

You foolish Galatians! Who has bewitched you?
Before your very eyes Jesus Christ was clearly por-
trayed as crucified....Did you receive the Spirit by the
works of the law, or by believing what you heard?
—GALATIANS 3:1–3

How do you feel when you are lied to or deceived? Sometimes we even lie to ourselves or hear only what we want
to, knowing it is not really true. The American Academy of
Pediatrics recently discussed how to deal with childhood obesity...and recommended *drugs!*[1] This is an example of how
deception can work. We don't want to be told that we are at
fault, made a mistake, or were fooled or deceived. When we
have health concerns, we rarely take responsibility for our
lifestyles or habits. We find someone to tell us what pill to
take. We allow ourselves to be deceived. Like the Galatians,
we can see the truth (in their case, about Christ's resurrection) and still be deceived. Take this scripture as a warning.

TAKE HEART

Do you seek out teaching that makes you feel better without
dealing with tough issues? The devil loves to deceive and confuse us. Resist his ways. Do not fall for his tricks.

TAKE ACTION

Review any areas of your life where you have let things slide or
bought into the world's wisdom. Stay the course of truth, even
when it is difficult.

KNOWN BY GOD

*Formerly, when you did not know God, you were slaves
to those who by nature are not gods. But now that you
know God—or rather are known by God—how is it that
you are turning back to those weak and miserable forces?
Do you wish to be enslaved by them all over again?*
—GALATIANS 4:8–9

W E ARE ALL born into Adam's sin, enslaved to the world. But through God's Son, we can be saved and set free. We come into relationship with God and are known by Him. It is truly amazing, and I would suggest it is one of the greatest miracles. If you are reading this and you are one of those known by God, celebrate! Give thanks.

However, here is something equally remarkable: even after this amazing rescue we still fall for the devil's traps. This scripture is a warning from Paul. Cling to Jesus, the One who saved us and set us free!

TAKE HEART

Have you ever fallen back into sin? Are you in that season now? Today is the day to return!

TAKE ACTION

Identify areas of your life where you are out of alignment. Take them to Jesus. Repent. And start anew.

FREEDOM

It is for freedom that Christ has set us free. Stand firm, then, and
do not let yourselves be burdened again by a yoke of slavery.
—GALATIANS 5:1

IF YOU STRUGGLE with issues such as addiction, emotional
health, or habitual sin, this scripture is for you! For freedom
Christ has set us free; stand firm, and do not submit again to
the yoke of slavery.

Many times when we listen to testimonies of people who
have been saved by Jesus, we hear some version of *freedom—*
from sin, addiction, fear, infirmity, etc. Jesus is a chain breaker.
The ultimate freedom is found in and through Him.

Now if you struggle and you don't feel free, again you are
not alone. Keep pressing into the promises of God. Keep
praying; keep reading His Word; keep worshipping. He is the
only one who can truly set you *free.*

TAKE HEART

Have you experienced freedom in Christ?

TAKE ACTION

Where do you not feel free? Surrender this area to Christ.

IS YOUR FISHBOWL DIRTY?

A little yeast works through the whole batch of dough.
—GALATIANS 5:9

IMAGINE A FISH in a fishbowl. If the fish lives in dirty water, what will happen? Yes, the fish will "get sick." Is the fish sick because it has bad fish DNA? Should we sprinkle on some "fishy" drugs to treat him? Or should we just clean the water? And if we clean the water, what will likely happen to the fish? Yes, he will heal and get healthier! It is a fish miracle!

TAKE HEART

Why do we understand this with fish and not ourselves? How is your fishbowl looking?

TAKE ACTION

Write down all the things that make up the fishbowl of your life—social life, work, stress, food, exercise, drugs, sleep, and so on. Look at the list. How does your fishbowl look? What do you need to change?

WISE WORDS

*You, my brothers and sisters, were called to be
free. But do not use your freedom to indulge the
flesh; rather, serve one another humbly in love.*
—GALATIANS 5:13

Do NOT USE your freedom to indulge in a sinful manner,
but serve one another in love. Sometimes we tend to take
Christ's love, grace, and freedom for granted. We abuse these
gifts and pervert them. We think, "Christ is cool with me. I
can do whatever I want and He will forgive me." These are not
the thoughts of a new creation or a transformed heart. They
are the thoughts of a still selfish, flesh-filled human.

Suppose you were in prison and were set free. Yes, you
would be free, but if you walked across the street and robbed
the store, you would be going back to jail. Use your freedom
for good, for love.

TAKE HEART

When you sin, what do you think God thinks? What do the
Scriptures say about how He feels about sin?

TAKE ACTION

Reflect on how you are using your freedom. Are there areas
where you are taking advantage of it?

Day 247

LIFE BY THE SPIRIT

*But the fruit of the Spirit is love, joy, peace, forbear-
ance, kindness, goodness, faithfulness, gentleness and
self-control. Against such things there is no law.*
—GALATIANS 5:22–23

IN TODAY'S STRESSFUL, fallen world, we can often get overcome by the endless stream of things we hear and see to
get worried about. It affects us. I love this passage because
it shows us what our lives should look like when we are
filled with the Spirit. As you read this list again, ask yourself
whether you reflect these gifts: love, joy, peace, forbearance
(patience), kindness, goodness, faithfulness, gentleness, and
self-control.

TAKE HEART

How are you looking? Do you reflect these fruits of the Spirit?
What areas do you need to improve?

TAKE ACTION

Pick one area. Take it to the Lord and ask for His help.

Day 248
TODAY IS THE DAY!

*Each one should test their own actions. Then they
can take pride in themselves alone, without com-
paring themselves to someone else.*
—GALATIANS 6:4

A N OLD ADAGE says, "The best time to plant a tree was
thirty years ago. The second-best time is today." Sometimes we say, "Well, it is too late." The great news is that it is
never too late to start doing the next right thing. There are
always benefits to caring for the body God gave you! Start
today!

TAKE HEART

Ask yourself if today is the day to improve your health journey.
Are you ready to start?

TAKE ACTION

Do something today to start. Have a glass of water. Do a push-
up. Go on a walk!

Day 249
DO NOT GROW WEARY IN DOING GOOD WORK

Let us not become weary in doing good, for at the proper time we will reap a harvest if we do not give up.
—GALATIANS 6:9

SOMETIMES WE FEEL like it's too hard. We get tired; we get to the end of our ropes; we don't seem to get the results we wanted; we stumble; we doubt; we grow weary. God knows this. God speaks to this.

Jesus experienced temptation when He walked the earth as a man, and He spoke into this. He implores us. He warns us; He contends for our hearts. He knows this will come up. He knows it won't be easy. He simply says to not grow weary in doing good work. It's worth it. Stay the course, even when it doesn't seem to be working—especially then. Stay focused on the good, on God. Don't give in; run the race and fight the good fight.

TAKE HEART

Have you had seasons of weariness? Are you in one now? What is Jesus saying to you?

TAKE ACTION

Do the next right thing. And then the next. One day at a time, one step at a time.

Day 250

THE GOSPEL: REMEMBER *WHO* AND *WHOSE* YOU ARE

*For [God] chose us in him before the creation of the world
to be holy and blameless in his sight. In love he predestined
us for adoption to sonship through Jesus Christ, in accordance with his pleasure and will—to the praise of his glorious
grace, which he has freely given us in the One he loves.*
—EPHESIANS 1:4–6

EPHESIANS 1 IS powerful. Sometimes, to know where you're going, you need to know where you have been. The first thing we must remember is God "chose us in him before the creation of the world." We often say we "choose to follow God." But the truth is, He chose us. It's important we remember that to keep our perspective accurate and to stay humble. He pre-destined us to be adopted as His children, to receive His grace, which He freely gives us.

Just sit and think about this. He—God, the King of the universe—chose *you*! It's not the other way around. He deserves all the glory. And after He chose you, you became a son or daughter of the King. Wow!

TAKE HEART

Does this truth overwhelm your heart? Who are we to deserve such love and grace?

TAKE ACTION

Reflect on how you view your role in salvation. Have you had it backward? Use this scripture to reorient to the truth.

Day 251

FOR THE PRAISE OF HIS GLORY

In him we were also chosen, having been predestined
according to the plan of him who works out everything in con-
formity with the purpose of his will, in order that we, who
were the first to put our hope in Christ, might be for the praise
of his glory. And you also were included in Christ when you
heard the message of truth, the gospel of your salvation.
—EPHESIANS 1:11–13

MUCH OF TODAY's culture tends to glorify man more than God. This passage reminds us of the proper perspective. We were chosen by God to find hope in Christ, for His praise and glory. Not for us. Not for ourselves. The call is for us to pour out our lives as living sacrifices that honor and glorify God, not for God to glorify us. As if He is here to make much of us—if we believe that perversion, we will feel like we got the short end of the stick. This leads to frustration, weariness, and complaining. We must choose the Word, seek the mercies of God, etc. Our perspective matters.

TAKE HEART

Do you spend more time complaining to God about what you think you want or need than glorifying and praising God?

TAKE ACTION

This could be a profound shift for you. Really meditate on what God is saying here.

EVEN WHEN WE WERE DEAD IN OUR TRANSGRESSIONS

You were dead in your transgressions and sins, in which you used to live when you followed the ways of this world....All of us also lived among them at one time, gratifying the cravings of our flesh and following its desires and thoughts. Like the rest, we were by nature deserving of wrath. But because of his great love for us, God, who is rich in mercy, made us alive with Christ even when we were dead in transgressions.
—EPHESIANS 2:1–5

EPHESIANS IS LIKE a stiff cup of coffee reminding us exactly who Christ is, why He came, and why He chose us. This scripture lays out a crucial point: Christ died for us even while we were dead in our transgressions. He saw the potential, but He knew He would have to do all the work. We were helpless. We were goners. We were dead.

But God rescued us from ourselves. We had nothing to do with it. He chose *us*! If you know God, it's not because of anything you did. You did not choose Him. He chose you before the creation of the earth. *Thank You, Jesus.*

TAKE HEART

How grateful would you be if you needed an organ to live and someone donated one? Through that person's death, you lived.

TAKE ACTION

Continue to meditate on what Christ did for you. Don't stop until you are overwhelmed by His grace.

SAVED BY GRACE—GOD'S GIFT

*For it is by grace you have been saved, through
faith—and this is not from yourselves, it is the gift of
God—not by works, so that no one can boast.*
—Ephesians 2:8–9

MANY SALVATION STORIES seem to be some version of "I
went to church. I said a prayer and accepted Jesus into
my heart." I know this is an oversimplification, but it's important that we discuss this.

It's God's grace that saved you—period. It's a gift you did
not deserve. At all. Period. Until we remove any work and
pride from our experience of salvation, we will always have
a root in our hearts that says we had something to do with it.

We think that we sat and listened and that, because we
are so smart, *we* decided to allow Jesus to save us! Wow, the
hubris.

TAKE HEART

Think back to your salvation experience. How do you
remember it? How do you talk about it? Do you need to
renew it?

TAKE ACTION

Be intentional about how you describe being saved. Many
believers started off with the wrong perspective. Review and
repent as needed.

GOD PREPARED BEFOREHAND

For we are God's handiwork, created in Christ Jesus to do good works, which God prepared in advance for us to do.
—EPHESIANS 2:10

THIS SECTION OF Scriptures we have been discussing is so powerful. If you struggle with identity or God's love, grace, and mercy to you, these are critical verses for you.

You are His handiwork. Pause. Think through this. You were made by God. *Mind blown.* But it goes on and says He created us to do good works that He prepared beforehand.

God has a very specific plan and purpose for you through Christ. If you ever feel that your life doesn't matter, you're disagreeing with God. He made you in His image and laid out good works for you to do. Get after it!

TAKE HEART

Do you believe this about yourself or God?

TAKE ACTION

What "good works" do you think God has for you? Look at your history. List those things you feel God prepared for you.

BLOOD

*But now in Christ Jesus you who once were far away
have been brought near by the blood of Christ.*
—EPHESIANS 2:13

THERE IS SOMETHING about the blood of Jesus. It is amazing how our blood washes through the organs and tissues of our bodies, bringing in oxygen and nutrition and carrying away waste. It is also incredible how our blood cells are constantly *renewing*! And when you truly understand what the blood of Jesus did for you, you will never be the same.

TAKE HEART

Take one minute and feel your heartbeat. Jesus is sovereign over every one of those heartbeats. Oh how He loves you.

TAKE ACTION

Take Communion today. Really think about the blood that Christ shed for you.

Day 256

A POWERFUL PRAYER

I pray that out of [the Father's] glorious riches he may strengthen
you with power through his Spirit in your inner being, so that
Christ may dwell in your hearts through faith. And I pray that
you, being rooted and established in love, may have power...
to grasp how wide and long and high and deep is the love of
Christ, and to know this love that surpasses knowledge—that
you may be filled to the measure of all the fullness of God. Now
to him who is able to do immeasurably more than all we ask
or imagine, according to his power that is at work within us...
—EPHESIANS 3:16–20

THESE VERSES ABOUT God's power and majesty can set
you free! *Christ dwells* in our hearts. His love surpasses
knowledge. Jesus' power at work within us can do more than
anything we can think or ask for! If this seems hard to grasp,
consider this: What if, every millisecond, you had to think
about the trillions of cells in your body? Or about your survival? About the survival of your kids or the eight billion
people worldwide? How about the stars, the planets' orbits,
etc.? When we realize the majesty of God, residing in us and
in our hearts, it's overwhelming.

TAKE HEART

How do you feel when you read this? Thankful? Overwhelmed?

TAKE ACTION

Pray this scripture daily for seven days. Write these verses on
your heart.

256   *DESIGNED TO HEAL*

Day 257

WORTHY OF THE CALL!

I...exhort you to walk in a manner worthy of the calling with which you were called. With all humility, meekness, and patience, bearing with one another in love...
—Ephesians 4:1–2, mev

God has a calling on your life. The Scriptures are very clear. He chose you, before creation, and He prepared good work for you. Now, you may say you don't know your calling, but that does not mean you don't have one. You have a calling. You have a calling *from God Himself*! What a humble honor.

So what does Paul tell us? "Walk in a manner worthy" of your calling. We play a role in this. We are not robots or puppets. God gives us free will. We need to show up and engage. Walk it out.

Take Heart

Are you living in a manner worthy of the calling on your life?

Take Action

If the answer above is *no*, what do you need to change? Start that process today.

A MEASURE OF GRACE

*But to each one of us grace has been
given as Christ apportioned it.*
—EPHESIANS 4:7

WE TEND TO compare our lives to others. We look around and see what others have and don't have, and it often makes us feel either bad or better about ourselves. But consider this: Christ has given *each one* of us a specific measure of grace based on His perfect perspective of what He has called us to do in our lives. Instead of focusing on what others seem to have or not have, let us focus on the *perfect* gifts given to us—for God's specific purposes!

TAKE HEART

Meditate on the powerful reality that God Himself, as He created you (before you were aware), knew exactly what amount of grace you would need. Just feel how powerful that is.

TAKE ACTION

If you find that you often compare yourself to others, anchor to these scriptures. Memorize them, and remind yourself that God *Himself* has perfectly equipped you with all the grace you need. And remember, His grace is sufficient.

GROW UP

*Then we will no longer be infants, tossed back and forth
by the waves, and blown here and there by every wind of
teaching and by the cunning and craftiness of people in their
deceitful scheming. Instead, speaking the truth in love, we
will grow to become in every respect the mature body of
him who is the head, that is, Christ. From him the whole body,
joined and held together by every supporting ligament, grows
and builds itself up in love, as each part does its work.*
—EPHESIANS 4:14–16

A S WE MATURE in our walks with and knowledge of Christ, *real, tangible* changes and fruits should be visible in our lives. We should no longer be "tossed back and forth." We should not fall so easily for the enemy's tricks. We should be growing up in Christ, and we should look more like Him every day. Some say that couples who have been together for several years often start to resemble each other. I'm not sure if this is true, but after years of intimacy with Jesus, we should very much look like Him.

TAKE HEART

Do you look more like Jesus than you did a year ago? Or did you just use Jesus as your "get out of hell" card and then went back to your life?

TAKE ACTION

Reflect on the last five years, one year, six months, six weeks. List the evidence of your maturity in Christ.

NEW LIFE

*They are...separated from the life of God because of...the hard-
ening of their hearts. Having lost all sensitivity, they...indulge
in every kind of impurity, and they are full of greed. That,
however, is not the way of life you learned...in accordance
with the truth that is in Jesus. You were taught, with regard
to your former way of life, to put off your old self, which is
being corrupted by its deceitful desires; to be made new in
the attitude of your minds; and to put on the new self, created to be like God in true righteousness and holiness.*
—EPHESIANS 4:18–24

WE HAVE BEEN walking through Ephesians, considering
the powerful gift of God's grace and His choosing to
save us, as well as the incredible calling and purpose He has
for you and me. Paul now goes after things a little harder. Basically, he implores us to put off our old selves and be renewed
in the spirit of our minds. "Put on the new self," created in the
likeness of God, in true righteousness and holiness.

Amazing, isn't it? This kind of reminds me of a pep talk
in the locker room. Paul's reminding us of who we are in
Christ—now go play and live that way!

TAKE HEART

Are there areas of your life that need renewal?

TAKE ACTION

List the areas where you are still living as your old self. Renew
your mind.

Day 261

RENEW YOUR MIND

And be renewed in the spirit of your mind.
—EPHESIANS 4:23, MEV

MANY PEOPLE ARE prescribed medications to deal with depression. Yet when these medications are compared with other treatments such as exercise or homeopathy, the prescription drugs are one of the least effective.[1] Several factors can influence our emotions. If you are struggling with depression, be sure you explore all the different options.

Treatments for Depression: Short-Term Outcomes[2]

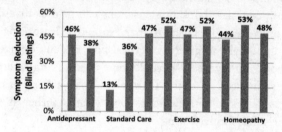

TAKE HEART

The chemical-imbalance theory of depression has never been proven.[3] Do you think people can heal from depression?

TAKE ACTION

Marketing has convinced us that the only way to treat depression is with medication—often forever. Research the many different options available, including diet, detox, exercise, and spiritual interventions such as prayer and Christian counseling.

Day 262
FORGIVENESS

*Be kind and compassionate to one another, forgiving
each other, just as in Christ God forgave you.*
—EPHESIANS 4:32

A T THE TIME of writing this devotional, I have worked
in the health-care field for about twenty years. If you
asked me to list some of the most powerful concepts relating
to healing and disease, I would include forgiveness near the
top. I have personally witnessed profound healings and break-
throughs when forgiveness is involved. I have also seen disease manifest from lack of forgiveness.

Now, countless books and sermons can help us dive deep
into forgiveness, but I want to make sure we at least bring this
topic up. Maybe forgiveness is the whole reason you needed
this book. Forgiveness—period. Some need to forgive others,
while some need to forgive themselves. Jesus already has. He
tells us very straightforwardly—*forgive* one another as God
in Christ has forgiven you.

TAKE HEART

What do you need to forgive? If this is an issue for you, I suggest you get some good faith-based books on forgiveness to
walk through.

TAKE ACTION

If you need to forgive others or yourself, there is no better
time than now.

BE IMITATORS OF CHRIST

Follow God's example, therefore, as dearly loved children and walk in the way of love, just as Christ loved us and gave himself up for us as a fragrant offering and sacrifice to God.
—EPHESIANS 5:1–2

WHEN WE ARE told to imitate Christ, what does that mean? Well, Paul tells us to (1) walk in love (2) as Christ did for us, (3) as a fragrant offering and sacrifice to God. We are to offer our lives as fragrant offerings and sacrifices to God from a place of love!

How are you doing? Do people describe you as an imitator of Christ? Is your life a living sacrifice to God?

Love is not passive or wimpy. It is intense. It is intentional. It is truthful. It is fearless. It is *all*-in.

TAKE HEART

Do you think Jesus is worth it? He thought you were!

TAKE ACTION

List the fears or roadblocks you feel are preventing you from imitating Christ. Take them to Christ.

Day 264
BE WISE

Be very careful, then, how you live—not as unwise
but as wise, making the most of every opportu-
nity, because the days are evil. Therefore do not be
foolish, but understand what the Lord's will is.
—EPHESIANS 5:15–17

THE SCRIPTURES SPEAK often of wisdom—the importance
of making sound decisions, counting the costs, and living
intentionally. They remind us that we reap what we sow, that
there is the law of cause and effect. Sometimes we act like
children emotionally and intellectually; we want to knowingly
sin or "do what everyone else is doing," but we don't want to
experience the consequences. That is not wisdom.

Paul also reminds us to make the most of every opportunity. Again, we can get lazy and want God to do it all. Yet we
are to run the race God has for us. We are called to be people
of passion, going after the good works and plans God has for
us. Be wise and go after life!

TAKE HEART

Do you value wisdom? Do you have a zest for fulfilling the
plans God has for you?

TAKE ACTION

List a couple of big decisions you may face in the future. What
does wisdom look like?

THE FULL ARMOR OF GOD

Finally, be strong in the Lord and in his mighty power. Put on the full armor of God, so that you can take your stand against the devil's schemes.
—EPHESIANS 6:10–11

WALKING OUT YOUR journey with the Lord is more like a battle than a stroll through the park. Countless metaphors about war, battle, and fighting are used in the Scriptures. The reason this is so critical is that it allows you to understand and be emotionally prepared for what is in store. Think of it this way: if someone asked you to go on a walk, but you didn't know it was a ten-mile hike up a mountain, you would likely not be prepared and be very frustrated during that experience. It would have been better to know it was a mountain hike so you could be mentally and physically prepared for it.

Many people have quit on their relationship with Jesus because it was harder than they thought it would be. They went to war without armor and got hurt. Armor up!

TAKE HEART

Do you understand we are in a battle? Would you say you and your family are prepared?

TAKE ACTION

Get prepared. Don't show up to a gunfight with a water gun.

PRAY IN THE SPIRIT

And pray in the Spirit on all occasions with all kinds of prayers and requests. With this in mind, be alert and always keep on praying for all the Lord's people.
—EPHESIANS 6:18

THERE IS A secret to find out how much you value and believe in the power of prayer. Want to know how? Reflect on the last few days. How much did you pray?

We are called to pray—and to have the Word on our minds and hearts—continually. Trying to go through life without being armored up and prayed up is very dangerous. You are allowing yourself to go into battle without your weapons. Prayer is how we do battle in the spiritual realm. Maybe you have forgotten about the power of prayer and have been trying to fight a spiritual battle with natural means. It doesn't work that way. Be armored up and prayed up constantly!

TAKE HEART

Reflect on your prayer life. Are you prayed up in all areas? How about your prayers for others?

TAKE ACTION

Get a book or two on prayer, or watch or listen to a few sermons on prayer. Go after prayer. Be a prayer warrior!

CARRY IT TO COMPLETION

...being confident of this, that he who began a good work in you will carry it on to completion until the day of Christ Jesus.
—PHILIPPIANS 1:6

THIS IS SUCH an encouraging scripture. If you ever think it's over, that you missed your chance with Jesus, that He forgot or gave up on you, this scripture cuts straight to the heart and tells you exactly how this ends. Remember, God saved you. You don't save yourself. He is the God of the universe, the Alpha and Omega. He will see that His plans in and for your life are carried to completion. Jesus never fails. You won't be the first to prove otherwise.

TAKE HEART

Are you confident in Christ's good works in your life? Do you feel Him working in you?

TAKE ACTION

Pray a prayer of thanksgiving right now for a God who never stops, never gives up, and never fails. Alleluia.

EVEN IN CHAINS

Now I want you to know, brothers and sisters, that what has happened to me has actually served to advance the gospel. As a result, it has become clear throughout the whole palace guard and to everyone else that I am in chains for Christ. And because of my chains, most of the brothers and sisters have become confident in the Lord and dare all the more to proclaim the gospel without fear.
—PHILIPPIANS 1:12–14

O NE REASON IT is powerful to read the Scriptures is that it gives us perspective. Paul's life definitely had many amazing peak moments, but I think very few reading this would truly want to walk in his shoes: multiple prison stunts, beatings, betrayal, thorn in his side, murder. Yet in the midst of this, *even while chained in prison*, Paul tells us his life still advanced the gospel. He says some were made aware of Christ and others were encouraged to share more boldly and courageously.

Remember, God will not be mocked. The gates of hell will not stop His church. Alleluia!

TAKE HEART

Do you feel that some circumstances have stopped you from living out God's plans and purposes in your life? Maybe you need a new perspective.

TAKE ACTION

Reflect on a time in your life that seemed terrible but now, looking back, you see what God did through it.

TO LIVE IS CHRIST, TO DIE IS GAIN

For to me, to live is Christ and to die is gain.
—PHILIPPIANS 1:21

THIS IS A mic-drop moment. It is a showstopping, game-changing perspective. Your entire life can be changed by the power of this one verse.

There are many insights this can give us. I will share a few, but it will likely touch your heart in a unique way. Here are a few considerations: (1) You woke up today—you are alive—because Christ allowed it and wants you to be on the planet today. The God of the universe desired to sustain you one more day. Amazing. (2) To die is to gain? Why? Because we are with Jesus for eternity, in heaven. When you no longer fear death, you are free! (3) When we realize that our lives are not our own, that we did not create ourselves and do not know when we will leave the earth, there is incredible freedom to live all out.

TAKE HEART

Are you afraid to die? Does that affect your decisions?

TAKE ACTION

List all the gains of death. Reflect on your fear and your perspective.

Day 270

DO NOTHING OUT OF
SELFISH AMBITION

*Do nothing out of selfish ambition or vain conceit. Rather, in
humility value others above yourselves, not looking to your
own interests but each of you to the interests of the others. In
your relationships with one another, have the same mindset as
Christ Jesus: Who...made himself nothing by taking the very
nature of a servant, being made in human likeness. And...he
humbled himself by becoming obedient to...death on a cross!*
—PHILIPPIANS 2:3–8

JESUS ALWAYS CUT straight to the heart. Paul's imploring
us to "do nothing out of selfish ambition" almost sounds
like heresy in today's "follow your bliss," "do you," "find your
truth," selfish culture. It's the complete opposite of all that.
Christ gave us the ultimate example.

I think the root of so much of our sin and pain is selfish
ambition. We want to be our own God, just like Adam and
Eve in the garden. We want to take credit. This is why it is so
critical that we die to self and to selfish ambition. Jesus is not
a genie here to grant your wishes. Die to self.

TAKE HEART

Do you consider yourself selfish? Think hard about this question. Maybe your selfishness shows up as safety, comfort, or
love for this world.

TAKE ACTION

If you discover selfishness, ask the Lord to heal your heart.

SHINE LIKE STARS

*Do everything without grumbling or arguing, so that
you may become blameless and pure, "children of God
without fault in a warped and crooked generation." Then
you will shine among them like stars in the sky.*
—PHILIPPIANS 2:14–15

I LOVE THIS DIRECT encouragement to us. Do everything without complaining or arguing so that you can shine like the stars in the universe. I have two children, and it sounds like a full miracle for them to go a day without arguing or complaining. Yet how many of us do the same thing in our spirits or with gossip or on social media? As the old saying goes, "Misery loves company." Are you miserable company? Paul is reminding us to keep from grumbling and complaining so we can shine our lights as blameless children of God, even in a depraved and crooked time.

TAKE HEART

Are you shining? Why or why not? Are you a complainer or grumbler?

TAKE ACTION

For one day, don't complain or argue. Give it a shot. I know you won't regret it.

THE SURPASSING GREATNESS
OF KNOWING CHRIST

*Whatever were gains to me I now consider loss for the sake
of Christ....I consider everything a loss because of the surpassing worth of knowing Christ Jesus my Lord....I consider
them garbage, that I may gain Christ and be found in him, not
having a righteousness of my own that comes from the law, but
that which is through faith in Christ....I want to know Christ.*
—PHILIPPIANS 3:7–10

IT'S FUNNY HOW excited people get when they meet a famous
person or go to a concert or a professional sports game. Idol
worship is alive and well. But it eats our souls and separates us
from the Father. Everything we have in life is nothing compared
to knowing Christ more. On one side you have everything in
the world, and on the other side you have Jesus. And Paul says
that whole side without Jesus is rubbish. Solomon, said to be
the "wisest man to ever live," indicated the same thing.

Jesus is enough. He's worth everything. Any perspective
less than this eats at our hearts. It creates envy, stress, worry,
and idols. The sooner we get that, the better.

TAKE HEART

Why do we get more excited about celebrities than God?

TAKE ACTION

List out everything in your life: kids, job, car, home, and so
on. Then on the other side write *Jesus*. He's better, and He
provided it all anyway!

STRAINING TOWARD WHAT IS AHEAD

*Brothers and sisters, I do not consider myself yet to
have taken hold of it. But one thing I do: Forgetting
what is behind and straining toward what is ahead, I
press on toward the goal to win the prize for which
God has called me heavenward in Christ Jesus.*
—PHILIPPIANS 3:13–14

I LOVE WITNESSING SIGNS and wonders and miracles of
God. It's incredible. But just as wonderful and special is
what Jesus does to our spirits when our hearts and minds are
healed. It's so amazing how much wisdom the Bible provides
for us about our minds and how we should posture our lives.

Depression, anxiety, sleep problems, and fatigue are
common health issues. Yet the Lord has much to say about
these. Although we all go through very real struggles, it is
critical we focus on the goodness of God and keep the faith.
Please do not misunderstand. Struggles with depression and
anxiety are very real, but let us never lose faith that God is for
us. When we are going through challenging times, it is often
easier to focus on our struggles than the goodness of God. It
is critical we have people in our lives speaking life into us.

TAKE HEART

Are you running your race? Do you look back too often?

TAKE ACTION

List things you feel are holding you back from the call or race
God has for you. Do you think they are bigger than God?

ESPECIALLY WHEN IT IS DIFFICULT

Become fellow imitators with me and observe those who walk according to our example. For many are walking in such a way that they are the enemies of the cross of Christ....Their destination is destruction, their god is their appetite, their glory is in their shame, their minds are set on earthly things.
—PHILIPPIANS 3:17–19, MEV

WHAT A SCRIPTURE. Although we may read this and think we are safe from the destruction, how many of us still have an appetite for the world? How many of us are consumed by sensual and worldly things? There is of course ample evidence of this inside and outside the church. Things we often call "blessings" can actually be idols that start to get between us and the Lord. Let us be so careful that we do not set our minds and hearts on earthly things.

TAKE HEART

When you reflect on your day and your choices, how much have you focused on earthly and fleshly things? Are your car, clothes, house, food, looks, and so on getting in the way of your relationship with Christ?

TAKE ACTION

Do something to shake yourself up a bit. Do you eat out too much? Shop too often? Spend a lot of time, money, and energy on your looks? For thirty days, don't go shopping. Don't eat out. Challenge yourself to focus on God instead.

PEACE THAT SURPASSES UNDERSTANDING

Rejoice in the Lord always. I will say it again: Rejoice! Let your gentleness be evident to all. The Lord is near. Do not be anxious about anything, but in every situation, by prayer and petition, with thanksgiving, present your requests to God. And the peace of God, which transcends all understanding, will guard your hearts and your minds in Christ Jesus.
—PHILIPPIANS 4:4–7

Do you find yourself worrying? Fearful of the future? Anxious? Maybe you don't use those words. Maybe you say you're "just realistic" or only want to "plan ahead," but really you are trying to build a life of comfort and safety. Well, here is some straightforward, holy scripture to reflect on: "Rejoice in the Lord *always*." If you are not rejoicing, start (even if you do not feel like it). Don't be anxious about *anything*. I know that's hard, which is why we must bring everything to God in prayer, praising and thanking Him. When we do, God will give us a supernatural peace.

Rejoice + Be anxious about nothing + Bring it to God = Total peace

TAKE HEART

Do you struggle with depression, fear, or anxiety? You don't have to. God is here to help!

TAKE ACTION

Commit this scripture to memory. Write it on your heart.

PRAY

Be anxious for nothing, but in everything, by prayer and supplication with gratitude, make your requests known to God.
—PHILIPPIANS 4:6, MEV

SEVERAL MEDICAL STUDIES and books have been written about the incredible power of prayer—specifically the *healing* power of prayer. When it comes to health and healing, we often think about what treatment we should do or what vitamin we should take, but let us never forget the most powerful tool we have: *prayer.*

Prayer is stronger than any drug, vaccine, or new fad diet. Prayer is real. Jesus showed us and reminded us constantly about taking everything to our Father in prayer. Prayer is not a last resort; it is our greatest *hope!*

TAKE HEART

How do you see prayer? Is prayer an important part of your daily walk? Do you pray for healing for yourself? For others?

TAKE ACTION

Make a prayer list. Keep it where you can see it often. Set reminders or alerts to remind you to pray. Pray for anything and everything. *Prayer works.*

AS A MAN THINKS...

*Finally, brothers, whatever things are true, what-
ever things are honest, whatever things are just, whatever things are pure, whatever things are lovely, whatever
things are of good report, if there is any virtue, and
if there is any praise, think on these things.*
—PHILIPPIANS 4:8, MEV

NINETY-FIVE PERCENT OF our behavior is automatic. There is a lot to say about the power of habit. Habits can work either for you or against you. The habit of prayer can transform your life. The habit of smoking can kill you.

Changing habits is challenging, and willpower alone often fails us. Include God and the Holy Spirit in the process of change. There are numerous studies that try to help us understand how long it takes to change our habits. Although there are many different ranges, two to six weeks is often the minimum amount of consistent time needed to disengage from a habit and/or commit to a new one.

TAKE HEART

What automatic habits do you have that are good for you? What are some that need to change?

TAKE ACTION

Pick one habit, and take it to God. Ask Him for direction and help through the process of change.

I CAN DO ALL THINGS THROUGH CHRIST WHO GIVES ME STRENGTH

*I know what it is to be in need, and I know what it is
to have plenty. I have learned the secret of being content in any and every situation, whether well fed
or hungry, whether living in plenty or in want. I can
do all this through him who gives me strength.*
—PHILIPPIANS 4:12–13

PAUL'S LETTER TO the Philippians ends with a bang. In a culture and time that are so wrapped up in materialism and "stuff," we would be well served to heed Paul's advice. He is talking about being content. Wouldn't that be a great place to live in your heart? Contentment. He says, "Listen, I have had a lot, and I have had nothing. I have learned that no matter what my life circumstances are, I'm content." And then he shares this amazing scripture: "I can do all this through him (Christ) who gives me strength!" Amazing. You are in big trouble if your God is only as good as your life circumstances. That's not how this works. I pray this scripture snaps open some of your heart and mind. He is enough.

TAKE HEART

Do you consider yourself content? Paul says you can be, and it can be *now*!

TAKE ACTION

Write what you think is preventing you from being content. Talk to God about it.

Day 279
LIVE A WORTHY LIFE

Live a life worthy of the Lord and please him in every way:
bearing fruit in every good work, growing in the knowledge
of God, being strengthened with all power according to his
glorious might so that you may have great endurance and
patience, and giving joyful thanks to the Father, who has quali-
fied you to share in the inheritance of his holy people in the
kingdom of light. For he has rescued us from the dominion of
darkness and brought us into the kingdom of the Son he loves.
—COLOSSIANS 1:10–13

IF ASKED WHETHER they want to live worthy lives, I think almost everyone would say yes. Now we could discuss what a "worthy" life is or isn't, but I think many people would also say something like "I want to, but it's hard. I get weary. I feel like I mess up." Yep. You are 100 percent correct. The only possible way we can do it is by being strengthened with God's power and glorious might. God *never, ever* intended for you to do this alone. That's exactly why He sent His Son and the Holy Spirit. Praise the Lord, you are not alone!

TAKE HEART

What do you do when you get weary or feel like you've failed? What does God say to do?

TAKE ACTION

You are not supposed to do this alone. We are colaborers with Christ. Ask the Lord to reveal an area He wants to partner with you on to change, and commit to responding to His leading.

JESUS HOLDS US ALL TOGETHER

He is before all things, and in him all things hold together.
—COLOSSIANS 1:17

Y OU MAY HAVE never heard of laminin. Laminin is a protein in our bodies. I just love how God sometimes leaves
little clues or insights that show His divine design. Here is the
amazing thing about laminin: it is in the shape of a cross! And
it is often described as the protein that "holds us together."

Jesus is what holds us together. The cross was God's grand
design for redemption and healing. *Jesus, we need You—in
every cell of our beings.*

TAKE HEART

What do you think about these amazing aspects of God's
design? What do they stir in your spirit?

TAKE ACTION

Right now, wherever you are, give thanks to God for the
divine design that is *you*. He even gives you the ability to give
Him thanks!

Day 281
CHRIST IN YOU, THE HOPE OF GLORY

*To them God would make known what is the glo-
rious riches of this mystery among the nations. It
is Christ in you, the hope of glory.*
—COLOSSIANS 1:27, MEV

A s I SIT at my table early in the morning, working on this,
writing these by hand as the Lord directs, I am overwhelmed by this powerful statement. It's a moment when you
get to really ask yourself what "Christ in you" means to you.

Think about this: Many Old Testament fathers of the faith
never experienced the Holy Spirit and Christ in them! That
was not available until Jesus' death and resurrection. You, as a
saved child of God, have Christ in you—and thus, the hope of
glory! Literally, you have the greatest, infinite hope and glory
inside you!

There is no possible excuse you could come up with, no
scenario, no trauma, no experience that could attack and
remove the hope of glory through Christ in you. You truly
have *zero* excuses to not have a glory-filled life—period.

TAKE HEART

Do you feel the weight of this scripture? The transforming
power and reality of this? Wow.

TAKE ACTION

No excuses. Recognize the Spirit of God, and live with the
reality of this hope and glory.

Day 282
NEED SOME GOOD ADVICE?

*So then, just as you received Christ Jesus as Lord, continue to
live your lives in him, rooted and built up in him, strengthened in
the faith as you were taught, and overflowing with thankfulness.*
—COLOSSIANS 2:6–7

MANY TIMES WHEN I'm talking to patients, they just want
the quick fix, the "hack," the easy way. Oftentimes, the
solution is simple—it's just something we don't want to do.

Want to lose weight? Move more and eat less.

Want to be on social media less? Cancel your accounts. Log
off.

Here Paul lays out a lifetime's worth of advice in one sentence: You have received Christ; now continue to live in Him,
be rooted and built up in Him, be strengthened in faith, and
overflow in thankfulness.

Pretty simple. Do that forever, and you will be fine.

TAKE HEART

Do you overcomplicate your relationship with Jesus? Do you
want Him and the world? Keep it simple.

TAKE ACTION

Reflect on your life and habits. What do you need to cut out?
Do it today.

Day 283
DON'T BE FOOLED

See to it that no one takes you captive through hollow and deceptive philosophy, which depends on human tradition and the elemental spiritual forces of this world rather than on Christ.
—COLOSSIANS 2:8

How EASY IT can be to be deceived and captivated by the ways of this world. We often look back at Adam and Eve and can't believe they fell for the devil's tricks. But the truth is, we can and still do the same. We make idols out of people, and we seek man's ways rather than Christ's ways. *Oh, Lord, have mercy on us. Forgive our shallow ways. We need You only.* Today weak teaching, self-glorifying lifestyles, and fleshly addiction opportunities abound. *Lord, we need You.*

TAKE HEART

When you look at people you admire, books you read, or podcasts you listen to, do you put more weight on those than on Christ?

TAKE ACTION

Live like your life depends on Christ—because it does.

EYES UP

Since, then, you have been raised with Christ, set your hearts on things above, where Christ is, seated at the right hand of God.
—COLOSSIANS 3:1

HAVE YOU EVER been walking down the road with your head down and hit your head on something like a sign or a tree? Had you been looking up, you would have seen it. In this scripture we are counseled that since we have been raised with Christ, we are to set our hearts and minds on things *above*, not earthly things. What a powerful reminder we need almost daily.

Let us be a people who stay focused on the things that truly matter—the things of God and heaven and His kingdom. Let us lose our taste for the things of the world.

TAKE HEART

Where are your eyes? Where are you focused: on God or man?

TAKE ACTION

List five things of this world that take a lot of your focus. They can be "good" things. How can you orient them toward God? If you cannot, some may need to go.

WHAT NEEDS TO DIE?

*Put to death, therefore, whatever belongs to your earthly
nature: sexual immorality, impurity, lust, evil desires and greed,
which is idolatry....You used to walk in these ways, in the life
you once lived. But now you must also rid yourselves of all...
anger, rage, malice, slander, and filthy language from your
lips. Do not lie to each other, since you have taken off your
old self with its practices and have put on the new self, which
is being renewed in knowledge in the image of its Creator.*
—COLOSSIANS 3:5–10

AGAIN, BACK TO the basics. Sin kills and destroys and separates us from God. The only way out is to put to death the
earthly, fleshly things that can consume our hearts. Paul lists
many here. Reread the list. What hits you? What areas do you
battle? Greed, lust, anger, filthy language? These are of the old
man. Time for a *new man*, a *godly* man. Put the old things to
death. Kill them before they kill you. This is not a game. This
is not a metaphor. The wages of sin are death. The cross allows
us to be free from sin.

TAKE HEART

Are you a slave to sin? Are you ready to be free?

TAKE ACTION

Get on your knees or face and cry out to the Lord. Ask Him
to show you and strengthen you to kill and prune the fleshly
things that need to die. Press in. Go for it. Go after it.

PEACE OF CHRIST

*Let the peace of Christ rule in your hearts, since as members of
one body you were called to peace. And be thankful....And
whatever you do, whether in word or deed, do it all in the name
of the Lord Jesus, giving thanks to God the Father through him.*
—COLOSSIANS 3:15–17

W E ALL SAY we want peace—in our world, our nation, our
cities, our houses, and our hearts. But there is only one
way to true and lasting peace: Christ.

We try so many other things to fill the void, to give us an
illusion of peace. We try laws, politics, materialism, divorce,
drugs, alcohol, Netflix, social media, work. We try almost
everything but Jesus. And we wonder. Sometimes, our
behavior reminds me of spoiled little kids who are never satisfied, always wanting the next thing or just a little more. Jesus
is the only thing that fills the void forever. True and lasting
peace is found with Him. "Whatever you do...do it all in the
name of Lord Jesus." Give thanks.

TAKE HEART

What things do you go to in order to get peace? How does it
work?

TAKE ACTION

Try Jesus. He knows you better than you know yourself. Let
the Prince of Peace bring peace.

Day 287
WORK FOR THE LORD

*Whatever you do, work at it with all your heart, as
working for the Lord, not for human masters, since you
know that you will receive an inheritance from the Lord
as a reward. It is the Lord Christ you are serving.*
—COLOSSIANS 3:23–24

ONE OF THE most common causes of stress is the work-
place. It is almost so commonplace now that most just
go along with it as helpless, hopeless victims. Yet again the
Scriptures give us a powerful perspective shift: *Whatever you
do, do it with all your heart* as working for the Lord.

Mic drop.

Do it unto the Lord. See your work—no matter what it is—
as an act of worship for the Lord.

Amazing, right? This perspective can shift everything for
you.

TAKE HEART

How can you reframe work and stress to help you have a better
perspective? Do you see your works as worship to the Lord?

TAKE ACTION

Don't let the enemy steal this time. Many of us spend most of
our days working somewhere. Let it be worship.

SEASONED WITH SALT

*Be wise in the way you act toward outsiders; make
the most of every opportunity. Let your conversation be always full of grace, seasoned with salt, so
that you may know how to answer everyone.*
—COLOSSIANS 4:5–6

HAVE YOU EVER sat down for a meal that looked great, but
after your first bite you knew it was missing something?
It needed to be seasoned. It needed some salt, some flavor.

This is part of the call of a Christian life. We are often so
busy worrying and complaining about how Christians are
treated or talked about, but this passage flips that on its head.
The responsibility of how we act toward others is 100 percent
on us, not them. We are to bring our best to conversations,
ready for any questions, full of grace and salt. What incredible advice that really stirs us outside ourselves and reminds
us to think about others and be a blessing to them. Amazing.

TAKE HEART

Is this how you think about talking to others, especially "outsiders"? Or do you often judge and try to answer too quickly?

TAKE ACTION

Today, while in conversation, be mindful about this advice.
While engaging, be salty and intentional!

FAITH, HOPE, AND LOVE

We remember before our God and Father your work pro-
duced by faith, your labor prompted by love, and your
endurance inspired by hope in our Lord Jesus Christ.
—1 THESSALONIANS 1:3

W E OFTEN TAKE credit for things that are not ours to take credit for. This verse is a powerful reminder of how God gives us everything. Here are the three great insights: (1) The good "work" we do was produced by *faith*, not us. (2) Our "labor" was not prompted by us; it was prompted by *love*. (3) Our endurance is inspired by *hope* in Jesus Christ. It's so crucial we understand the subtle nuance of taking credit for something Jesus allows us to do. He gives us faith, hope, and love, and out of those gifts we can take action.

TAKE HEART

Reflect on areas where you are taking credit. Do you use terms like *self-made* or say "Look what I did"? How we speak reveals our hearts.

TAKE ACTION

Look at all the things on your calendar today. Think about how God allows you to do those. If you work out, consider that God provided the body and mindset to do that. If you have a job, are married, or have children, the Lord provided all that. Thank Him.

DO NOT PUT OUT THE SPIRIT'S FIRE

Do not quench the Spirit.
—1 THESSALONIANS 5:19

W HAT A POWERFUL line. Remember, the God that is in you is the same God who hung the stars, hears every prayer, can do any sign or wonder, and died and forgave your sins. He is a mighty, powerful, majestic God. However, sometimes we "put Him in a box" because He makes us uncomfortable. He gives us gifts. He speaks to our hearts. He prompts us to take action. We need His Word and know we need to obey. But here we are reminded to not put out the Spirit's fire. If you feel stuck in life, if you feel you're going through the motions, a good heart check is to see whether you have stopped following the Spirit.

TAKE HEART

Are you sensitive to the Spirit? Do you hear the voice of the Good Shepherd? Do you obey?

TAKE ACTION

Today, pray. Ask God what He wants to say to you. Then *take action* on His response.

TEST EVERYTHING

But test them all; hold on to what is
good, reject every kind of evil.
—1 Thessalonians 5:21–22

Have you ever heard the saying "Ignorance is bliss"? Sometimes we hear or discover things we wish we hadn't. Maybe a favorite preacher has a moral failure; maybe a friend has a double life; maybe we learn that certain habits or perspectives we hold are sinful and we get convicted. We then have a decision to make: Are we going to change? Speak out? In these complicated times, we can get overwhelmed and stop testing things. This scripture warns us not to do that.

Test *everything*. Hold on to *good*. Avoid *evil*.

Take Heart

Do you follow these three great truths? Which one do you struggle with? Why?

Take Action

Think of areas where you don't test; you simply trust human wisdom. A recent example happened during COVID-19 where many people, out of fear and pressure, made decisions that they never tested. Repent of anything like that in your life.

THEY REFUSED TO LOVE TRUTH

...and all the ways that wickedness deceives those who are
perishing. They perish because they refused to love the
truth and so be saved. For this reason God sends them
a powerful delusion so that they will believe the lie.
—2 THESSALONIANS 2:10–11

"TRUTH SOUNDS LIKE hate to those who hate the truth." We all have friends or family who have not been saved. This can be one of the most challenging aspects of being in Christ. You may struggle with how to interact, how to navigate the relationships. This passage offers another perspective that may help.

God allows some who refuse truth to believe the lies of Satan. This can be hard to read when it describes people we love and care about, but it can also help explain some behaviors we see. When we, or anyone else, resist loving truth, we are now dancing with the enemy. We have opened ourselves to delusion. We must be on guard.

TAKE HEART

Do you have people in your life who hate the truth of Jesus? How do you generally respond?

TAKE ACTION

Thank God right now for the gift of faith, for not handing you over to the evil one.

GET BUSY

*We were not idle when we were with you, nor did we eat any-
one's food without paying for it. On the contrary, we worked
night and day, laboring and toiling so that we would not
be a burden to any of you. We did this...to offer ourselves
as a model for you to imitate...."The one who is unwilling to
work shall not eat." We hear that some among you are idle
and disruptive. They are not busy; they are busybodies. Such
people we command...to settle down and earn the food
they eat. And as for you...never tire of doing what is good.*
—2 Thessalonians 3:7–13

AGAIN, YOU HAVE to appreciate the practical teachings in the
Bible. Here Paul emphasizes the importance of work and
a good work ethic. Over time, especially during the pandemic,
we have witnessed a shift in people having a desire to work. It's
a slippery slope. Idle time is not a good thing. We need to earn
a living, and we need to serve others in the marketplace. The
Scriptures are very clear about this. We are not to be lazy. We
are to be productive citizens—not for the world's rat race but
for God! We are to reflect God well. Work is good.

TAKE HEART

How do you view work? When you have too much time, how
do you do?

TAKE ACTION

Reflect on time in relation to your life. How do you manage
idle time?

CHRIST JESUS CAME TO SAVE SINNERS

*I urge, then, first of all, that petitions, prayers, intercession
and thanksgiving be made for all people....This is good, and
pleases God our Savior, who wants all people to be saved
and to come to a knowledge of the truth. For there is one
God and one mediator between God and mankind, the man
Christ Jesus, who gave himself as a ransom for all people.*
—1 TIMOTHY 2:1-7

PAUL CUTS RIGHT to the chase. Jesus is the one who does
the saving, not us. Christ died for us. The price Christ
paid for Paul (a big sinner, he says) is an example of the Lord's
mercy and patience. Paul was not looking for God when he
was wiped out by the Lord.

We often get this backward. We think we choose to be
saved. Nope. He saves us. We cannot, under any circumstances, save ourselves. We are the created; He is the Creator.
He is God. We are not. It is one of the most humbling aspects
of the gospel. May it forever keep us on our knees in gratitude
and thanksgiving to Him.

TAKE HEART

Have you thanked Jesus today for saving you? You didn't
choose Him; He chose you!

TAKE ACTION

List all your past sins—the things you have done. Stare at that
list. God sent His Son to die for that list, to save you! Amazing.

MANAGE YOUR FAMILY

*If anyone does not know how to manage his own
family, how can he take care of God's church?*
—1 Timothy 3:5

THIS IS SOME strong teaching. Now this particular verse is giving some requirements for deacons of the church, but it is important for us all to consider. We are called to manage our families well. If we are unable to manage our families, we are not qualified to manage anything in the church.

This does not mean our families are to be idols or an excuse not to serve others or the church. It means we are called to be good stewards. "Whoever can be trusted with very little can also be trusted with much" (Luke 16:10). Be aware. We all know that managing a family is challenging. But take responsibility for your family and yourself. It's important.

TAKE HEART

Are you taking your family responsibility seriously? Are you engaged with them? Stewarding your family well? What areas need work?

TAKE ACTION

Sometimes we want to be involved in other things to avoid family stress. It never works. Get in the game in your house.

SOME WILL ABANDON THE FAITH

*The Spirit clearly says that in later times some will abandon
the faith and follow deceiving spirits and things taught by
demons. Such teachings come through hypocritical liars,
whose consciences have been seared as with a hot iron.*
—1 Timothy 4:1–2

This is a warning from the Holy Spirit to us and for us.
"In later times some will abandon the faith and follow
deceiving spirits." This is concerning. What prevents *you*
from being one of them? I have a family member that this
happened to. It's very difficult to watch and witness and even
to understand.

We must remember, the enemy is always looking for ways
to tempt, destroy, and kill. We must stay on guard for ourselves, our families, and others. We are told to contend for
and to renew our minds daily. Don't coast. Don't get lazy in
your faith. Press in, and finish the race.

TAKE HEART

Have you ever known people who abandoned their faith?
When you reflect, can you see when they slipped?

TAKE ACTION

Be ready, on guard. Stay in the Word. Stay in prayer. Stay connected. We are in a battle. Don't get distracted or off-track.

GODLINESS WITH CONTENTMENT

*But godliness with contentment is great gain. For we brought
nothing into the world, and we can take nothing out of it. But
if we have food and clothing, we will be content with that.
Those who want to get rich fall into temptation and a trap
and into many foolish and harmful desires that plunge people
into ruin and destruction. For the love of money is a root of
all kinds of evil. Some people, eager for money, have wan-
dered from the faith and pierced themselves with many griefs.*
—1 TIMOTHY 6:6–10

CHASING THE THINGS of this world often causes us much
strife, stress, and problems. Paul is laying out some good
life principles that we should heed. First he tells us to be content in being godly. At times people wrongly perceive that
being godly is restrictive, but nothing could be further from
the truth. God's ways are for our benefit.

Paul also warns us about desiring money, telling us that
the *love* of money is the root of many evils. He encourages us
to be content with food and clothing. Look how far we have
drifted. So many people have discontented lives because the
world tells them to want more. God says, "Be careful!"

TAKE HEART

Have you seen the love of money ruin lives? Do you consider
yourself content?

TAKE ACTION

Reflect on what you are striving for. Are you content?

Day 298

FIGHT THE GOOD FIGHT OF FAITH

*Fight the good fight of the faith. Take hold of the eternal
life to which you were called when you made your
good confession in the presence of many witnesses.*
—1 TIMOTHY 6:12

WE ALL WANT to live a life that matters, a life with meaning. Paul tells us what that looks like: "Fight the good fight of faith." What an interesting thought—the good fight of faith. It reminds us that walking and living in faith are not easy. We must fight and contend for it, and it's a good and worthy fight.

What happens if we stop fighting for our faith? Over time we will lose our faith, which leads to backsliding—slipping into the ways of the world, making bad decisions due to our lack of faith.

TAKE HEART

Are you fighting the good fight? How's it going?

TAKE ACTION

List some ways you can fight for your faith, such as praying, reading the Word of God, worshipping, and making a sacrifice such as fasting.

DESIGNED TO HEAL

Day 299

A WARNING TO THE RICH

Command those who are rich in this present world not to be arrogant nor to put their hope in wealth, which is so uncertain, but to put their hope in God, who richly provides us with everything for our enjoyment. Command them to do good, to be rich in good deeds, and to be generous and willing to share. In this way they will lay up treasure for themselves as a firm foundation for the coming age, so that they may take hold of the life that is truly life.
—1 TIMOTHY 6:17–19

I'M SURE YOU have seen the statistics telling us that, even though we don't believe it, many of us are rich compared to most of the rest of the world. If you have a next meal and some change in your pocket, you're doing okay. Paul reminds us to not put our hope in wealth because it is uncertain. Instead we are to put our hope in God, who "richly provides" our every need. He also implores us to be generous and willing to share. By doing this, we will store treasures in heaven and take hold of what life truly is. Let us not be controlled by money.

TAKE HEART

Do you think a lot about money? Do you consider yourself rich? Are you generous?

TAKE ACTION

Go give today. Increase your giving at church. Help someone. It is good not just for them but also for you.

A SPIRIT OF POWER

For the Spirit God gave us does not make us timid,
but gives us power, love and self-discipline.
—2 TIMOTHY 1:7

A s CHILDREN OF God, filled with the Holy Spirit, we are
called to live a bold life. The Spirit enables us to live a life
of power, love, and self-discipline.

Do not live timid lives. Jesus was bold. Paul was bold. Peter
was bold. And Jesus tells us to not hide our light under a bowl
but to be salt and light (Matt. 5:13–16). As you pour out your
life as an offering to God, those around you will notice. It will
encourage and bless them.

TAKE HEART

Are you living a life of power in Christ? Why or why not?

TAKE ACTION

Do one thing for Jesus today. Share the gospel, invite someone
to church, talk to a stranger, volunteer, etc. Just do something
in the name of Jesus.

Day 301
FLEE EVIL DESIRES OF YOUTH

Flee the evil desires of youth and pursue righteousness, faith, love and peace, along with those who call on the Lord out of a pure heart. Don't have anything to do with foolish and stupid arguments, because you know they produce quarrels. And the Lord's servant must not be quarrelsome but must be kind to everyone, able to teach, not resentful. Opponents must be gently instructed, in the hope that God will grant them repentance leading them to a knowledge of the truth.
—2 Timothy 2:22–25

BEFORE CHRIST SAVED us, many of us had built up a pretty consistent life of sin, so when we begin to flee, it can be a challenge. Paul is again (through the power of the Holy Spirit) giving out crucial advice to help us walk this life out. He also tells us to have nothing to do with "foolish and stupid arguments" that just lead to quarrels. What a great reminder. I reflect back on how often I have had stupid arguments that just led to more problems. We would be wise to heed this advice, even though it may seem difficult at first.

TAKE HEART

Do you flee evil? Do you engage in foolish arguments? What do you think Jesus would say?

TAKE ACTION

What is an area in life you need to flee from? Identify it, repent, and flee. If you need help, get it!

Day 302

PEOPLE WILL BE LOVERS OF THEMSELVES—SELFIE CULTURE

But mark this: There will be terrible times in the last days. People will be lovers of themselves, lovers of money, boastful, proud, abusive, disobedient to their parents, ungrateful, unholy, without love, unforgiving, slanderous, without self-control, brutal, not lovers of the good, treacherous, rash, conceited, lovers of pleasure rather than lovers of God—having a form of godliness but denying its power. Have nothing to do with such people.
—2 TIMOTHY 3:1–5

THIS IMPORTANT PASSAGE helps us see and better understand the times we are living in. Think of how valuable it is when a friend or family member with children offers wisdom that helps you navigate parenting your first one. Sometimes we look at everything going on in the world and become overwhelmed, confused, or anxious. But then we read scriptures like this and remember that this is no surprise to God at all. He knew this would happen. How are we to respond to people like those described here? Paul writes, "Have nothing to do" with them.

TAKE HEART

Are you being changed by culture, or are you changing culture? Are you spending a lot of time with people like those Paul described?

TAKE ACTION

Reflect on your close relationships. Are they healthy? Does anything need to change?

ALL SCRIPTURE IS GOD BREATHED

All Scripture is God-breathed and is useful for teaching, rebuking,
correcting and training in righteousness, so that the servant
of God may be thoroughly equipped for every good work.
—2 TIMOTHY 3:16–17

I HAVE HEARD THE Bible sometimes referred to as "God's little instruction book." But it is so much more than that. It is the living, "God-breathed" Word of God. It has the power to transform your life. Nothing replaces reading, studying, meditating on, and memorizing God's Word. Remember, it is literally the *Word of God*!

When you are reading the Bible, how are you viewing it? As just a book? Some good suggestions? Truth? History? It is critical we see the Word of God as the most powerful, divine, living, breathing document ever created. We expect it to speak into our hearts and the power of the Holy Spirit to transform us.

TAKE HEART

What is your favorite verse? Why? How does Scripture affect you?

TAKE ACTION

Subscribe to an app or email that gives you daily scriptures. It's best to read and meditate on them in the morning.

BUT I LIKE IT!

*For the time will come when people will not put up with
sound doctrine. Instead, to suit their own desires, they
will gather around them a great number of teachers to
say what their itching ears want to hear. They will turn
their ears away from the truth and turn aside to myths.*
—2 Timothy 4:3–4

I F THERE WAS one area of nutrition I would encourage more
people to focus on, it would be reduction of sugar consumption. Lots of research shows that sugar-intake increase has led
to so many diseases and health issues—from obesity and diabetes to even cancer, heart disease, and Alzheimer's. This is
mostly because sugar causes inflammation, and inflammation is related to almost all disease processes. You would do
yourself a favor to significantly reduce sugar intake.

Take Heart

Just because something tastes good does not mean it is good
for you. Are you addicted to sugar and carbs? Are you ready
to make a change?

Take Action

Look at one day of your sugar and carb intake. What can you
change?

POURED OUT

*For I am already being poured out like a drink offering, and
the time for my departure is near. I have fought the good fight,
I have finished the race, I have kept the faith. Now there is in
store for me the crown of righteousness, which the Lord, the
righteous Judge, will award to me on that day—and not only
to me, but also to all who have longed for his appearing.*
—2 TIMOTHY 4:6–8

I LOVE PAUL'S DESCRIPTION of his life: "being poured out like
a drink offering." This was a common way to honor God
in the Old Testament. The Israelites would pour out wine on
the altar, and the fragrance that went up was pleasing to God
(Num. 28:7–8). What a great metaphor and goal—that the
aroma of our lives would be pleasing to God!

Paul also says he has fought the good fight, kept the faith,
and finished the race. This is an inspiring testimony for all
of us. We are all able to do this. Be empowered by the Holy
Spirit. Pour out your life for Jesus. Offer it up as a living sacrifice for the Lord.

TAKE HEART

If today was your last day, would you be able to say what Paul
did?

TAKE ACTION

Journal how this verse makes you feel. What emotions does it
stir up? What needs to change?

AT ONE TIME, WE TOO WERE FOOLISH

*At one time we too were foolish, disobedient, deceived and
enslaved by all kinds of passions and pleasures. We lived in
malice and envy, being hated and hating one another. But when
the kindness and love of God our Savior appeared, he saved us.*
—Titus 3:3–5

SOMETIMES WE FORGET what our lives were like before we
were saved. It becomes easy for us to judge and condemn
others. As a matter of fact, this is what keeps so many away
from Jesus—the way "believers" act toward them. As time
goes by, we often forget that we don't and didn't save ourselves. We didn't choose Jesus; He saved us. He chose us. It
wasn't because of anything we did; that way, none of us can
boast. It is critical that we remember this.

TAKE HEART

Do you remember when Jesus saved you? Did you have anything to do with it? Do you find yourself judging others often?

TAKE ACTION

Why is it so hard for us to give God the glory and credit?
Share your testimony today, but when you do, be careful how
you say it. You didn't "accept" Jesus. He saved you.

REGENERATION

Not by works of righteousness which we have done,
but according to His mercy He saved us, through the
washing of rebirth and the renewal of the Holy Spirit,
—Titus 3:5, MEV

IN CASE YOU needed more good news about fasting and healing, consider this: A recent study showed that the pancreas (think, blood sugar, insulin, and diabetes) can regenerate during a type of fasting diet![1] How amazing! We often underappreciate the God-given healing capacity of the human body. Examples like this remind us that there may be divine approaches to healing diseases typically viewed as incurable.

TAKE HEART

Do you think the body God created is probably capable of healing more than we give it credit for? Do you think we should try more natural approaches to health?

TAKE ACTION

Make fasting a habit. Try different types of fasts and for different lengths of time—such as a water or juice fast for one day, three days, or ten days.

REFRESHED THE HEARTS

Your love has given me great joy and encouragement, because you, brother, have refreshed the hearts of the Lord's people.
—PHILEMON 7

SOMETIMES YOU READ a certain verse and it just touches your heart. Doesn't it sound amazing to have your heart refreshed? It kind of makes me think of a car wash that you take your dirty, dusty car through and it comes out sparkling clean.

But here is the part that really touches me: this refreshing came from the love Paul felt from his friend. The love the Holy Spirit allows us to provide and show others can refresh hearts. What an honor and responsibility.

TAKE HEART

Are you a heart refresher? When people meet and interact with you, do they feel refreshed?

TAKE ACTION

Ask one to three people whether you are refreshing to them. Think of people who are refreshing to you. What is it that refreshes you?

TESTIFIED BY SIGNS, WONDERS, AND MIRACLES

God also testified to it by signs, wonders and various miracles, and by gifts of the Holy Spirit distributed according to his will.
—HEBREWS 2:4

THIS IS A great passage of Scripture. God Himself testified to the truth Jesus spoke by displaying signs, wonders, and gifts of the Holy Spirit. Amazing!

Do you regularly experience signs, wonders, and miracles and a moving of the Holy Spirit? These should be regular occurrences for people filled with the Holy Spirit.

TAKE HEART

When is the last time you had a supernatural, Holy Spirit experience?

TAKE ACTION

Put yourself in an environment or situation to expect the supernatural. It is not weird or crazy; it's *God*.

Day 310

ARE YOU AFRAID OF DEATH?

Since the children have flesh and blood, he too shared in their humanity so that by his death he might break the power of him who holds the power of death—that is, the devil—and free those who all their lives were held in slavery by their fear of death.
—HEBREWS 2:14–15

YOU HAVE PROBABLY heard it said that people are more afraid of public speaking than of dying. Well, I doubt this is true. Many people still rank death as their top fear.[1] The pandemic revealed how much fear of death so many have. But this amazing scripture passage reminds us that Jesus took care of death for us. He freed us from slavery to the fear of death.

I used to be terribly afraid of death. I had a significant anxiety about it. My parents even took me to a counselor for help. Yet it wasn't until Jesus saved me that I was free from the slavery of fearing death.

TAKE HEART

Are you afraid of dying? Why? What do you think Jesus would say? What do you think would be different if you were free from that fear?

TAKE ACTION

If you fear death, remember, Christ died to set you free. Pray for that freedom.

Day 311
REST

There remains, then, a Sabbath-rest for the people
of God; for anyone who enters God's rest also rests
from their works, just as God did from his.
—HEBREWS 4:9–10

REST. SLEEP. SABBATH. Are you a person who gets enough sleep? Who gets too much sleep? The Scriptures are loaded with truths about the importance of rest, Sabbath, and the sacred pace of life. In today's culture we are so addicted to busy life that we have almost lost the appreciation for rest and sleep. So many health conditions can be caused or worsened by lack of proper rest and sleep. The average adult needs between seven and eight hours of sleep a night. How are you doing?

TAKE HEART

How's your sleep life? Do you get too much? Too little? What's the quality of your sleep? Is it sporadic? Drug-induced?

TAKE ACTION

Look at sleep like nutrition or fitness. Good sleep is as important as any of those other factors. Set some ground rules, and work hard at resting!

THE WORD OF GOD IS ALIVE

For the word of God is alive and active. Sharper than any double-edged sword, it penetrates even to dividing soul and spirit, joints and marrow; it judges the thoughts and attitudes of the heart. Nothing in all creation is hidden from God's sight. Everything is uncovered and laid bare before the eyes of him to whom we must give account.
—HEBREWS 4:12–13

THIS SCRIPTURE TELLS us how powerful the Word of God is. It is sharper than a two-edged sword. It pierces through to the soul and the spirit. And no one can hide from it. We will all give an account. There is truly nothing more powerful than God and His Word.

Sometimes we will say something like "I don't know what to do," or we read scripture and say we are not really "feeling it." Rest assured; it is working. Don't avoid using one of the most powerful tools you have—the Word of God.

TAKE HEART

Do you use Scripture as a weapon? Do you see it as powerful as a sword?

TAKE ACTION

What is an area of your life you need God in? Use Scripture to go after it.

APPROACH THE THRONE OF GRACE WITH CONFIDENCE

*Let us then approach God's throne of grace with
confidence, so that we may receive mercy and
find grace to help us in our time of need.*
—HEBREWS 4:16

HAVE YOU EVER struggled to ask for help in a time of need? Even when you knew there were people and places that could help you? If you are struggling, being tempted, or suffering in any way, let this scripture remind you that you can confidently go to Jesus. He understands everything you have experienced. He was fully God yet fully human like us. He wants you to come to His throne of grace and mercy.

Or maybe this is a better question: Why *not* come to Him? Are you ashamed? Is it that you don't want to bother him? Don't think you need Him? Don't want Him involved?

TAKE HEART

Do you go to God when you are struggling? Why or why not?

TAKE ACTION

What area of your life have you not taken to God's throne? Write it down. Take it to the Lord. Let Him help you, and give Him all the glory.

ARE YOU MATURE?

Therefore let us move beyond the elementary teachings about Christ and be taken forward to maturity, not laying again the foundation of repentance from acts that lead to death, and of faith in God, instruction about cleansing rites, the laying on of hands, the resurrection of the dead, and eternal judgment. And God permitting, we will do so.
—HEBREWS 6:1–3

Do you consider yourself mature? Have you learned the basics and foundation of a Christian life and Christ's teachings? Do you have an understanding of the gospel, salvation, sanctification, spiritual gifts, and the Holy Spirit? Or are you acting and living like a baby? The Scriptures use this metaphor a few times. It is always good to ask ourselves if we are maturing in Christ and His ways. We should yearn for maturity in Christ. Just like there is nothing funny or cool about an adult acting like a kid, it is essential in our walk with Christ that we are maturing, that we are "working out" our salvation and growing in Christ.

TAKE HEART

How "old" of a Christian are you? Are you still maturing?

TAKE ACTION

Have you stopped maturing or growing in any areas of your faith? List them out. Pray about them.

Day 315
FAITH

Now faith is confidence in what we hope for
and assurance about what we do not see. This
is what the ancients were commended for.
—HEBREWS 11:1–2

FAITH IS BEING sure of what's hoped for and certain of what we don't see. Faith is amazing. Jesus said faith can move mountains. He said by our faith we can be healed. Scripture also says we are saved by faith. Faith is not "wishful thinking." It is not having a positive attitude; it is not the "law of attraction." To have faith in the things of God and hope in the promises of God, we need to know what those are. This is crucial.

TAKE HEART

Do you know the specifics about what the Scriptures say, or do you just "believe in God"?

TAKE ACTION

Commit to daily reading of Scripture. Read the Bible from cover to cover, and put it into action.

FAITH, CONTINUED

*These were all commended for their faith, yet none
of them received what had been promised.*
—HEBREWS 11:39

HEBREW 11 IS an amazing chapter that lists fascinating
examples of faith from the past. It is an incredible
reminder of the power of faith, from the stories of Abel to
Noah, Abraham to Moses, the Israelites at the Red Sea to Jericho, and more. It is very inspiring to read.

The last line of this chapter is so powerful. It tells us that
even though all these were commended for their faith, none
of them received what was promised. God had planned something even better—Christ and His death and resurrection.
Do you realize we live on the other side of the cross? All the
examples of faith we read in Hebrews 11 never got to experience Christ's coming. We have. Yes, we need faith, but we
also have the benefit of the resurrection, and that changes
everything.

TAKE HEART

Have you ever thought of this before? All of these had faith in
the coming Messiah. Yet we get to read about it actually happening and receive the Holy Spirit in us.

TAKE ACTION

If you struggle with keeping the faith, keep reading Hebrews
over and over. It will encourage you.

Day 317
THE WEIGHT OF SIN

*Therefore, since we are encompassed with such a
great cloud of witnesses, let us also lay aside every
weight and the sin that so easily entangles us.*
—HEBREWS 12:1, MEV

A WAY TO THINK about your health is to see all the areas of your lifestyle as rocks that you put in a backpack. The more rocks—or the bigger the rocks—the heavier the backpack will be, and the more it will affect your overall health.

Some of us are carrying around loads of stress, poor foods, poor sleep, lack of exercise, and more. We need to lighten up our backpacks so we can run the race we are called to run.

TAKE HEART

We may never get rid of all the stress and rocks in our backpacks, but we need to regularly check our backpacks and see if we need to empty some things. How is your backpack doing?

TAKE ACTION

Pick one rock to work on. Take action. When the backpack gets lighter, everything feels better.

Day 318

RUN THE RACE

*Therefore, since we are surrounded by such a great
cloud of witnesses, let us throw off everything that hinders and the sin that so easily entangles. And let us
run with perseverance the race marked out for us.*
—Hebrews 12:1

THIS SCRIPTURE IS well known for a reason—it is powerful. It is a critical reminder to run the race God has called you to. But there are some key points we need to make sure we do not gloss over.

"We are surrounded by such a great cloud of witnesses"— we are not running this race alone, my friend. Look who has gone before us. And we have God, Jesus, and the Holy Spirit also. Be encouraged and be confident.

"Let us throw off everything that hinders and the sin that so easily entangles"—many of us are running the race, but we are not going as far or as fast as we could because we carry so much shame, guilt, and sin. It is more like we are limping and stumbling down the street. We must throw off the junk and *run* the race!

TAKE HEART

How is your race going?

TAKE ACTION

Remove the baggage and sin in your life. What do you need to get rid of so you can more effectively run your race?

Day 319
THE AUTHOR OF OUR FAITH

Let us look to Jesus, the author and finisher of our faith, who for the joy that was set before Him endured the cross, despising the shame, and is seated at the right hand of the throne of God.
—HEBREWS 12:2, MEV

HERE ARE THE latest health statistics for the United States: compared with other leading countries, we spend the most on health care, but we have the lowest life expectancy.[1] Now I am not the smartest guy in the room, but something does not seem to be working! This does not seem to be a good return on investment. Have you ever heard that the definition of *insanity* is doing the same thing over and over again and expecting a different result? We keep throwing more drugs, more vaccines, and more tests at the problem, and it is *getting worse*. Maybe the approach is the problem!

TAKE HEART

Does this surprise you? What can you do to improve your odds?

TAKE ACTION

The single biggest variable for your health and longevity is the daily choices you make. Do a review of your lifestyle. Are you on the right track? If not, get some help.

THE DISCIPLINE OF GOD

*Endure hardship as discipline; God is treating you as his chil-
dren. For what children are not disciplined by their father?
If you are not disciplined—and everyone undergoes discipline—then you are not legitimate, not true sons and daughters
at all. Moreover, we have all had human fathers who disciplined us and we respected them for it. How much more should
we submit to the Father of spirits and live! They disciplined
us for a little while as they thought best; but God disciplines
us for our good, in order that we may share in his holiness.*
—HEBREWS 12:7–10

N̲O ONE LIKES to be disciplined. But make no mistake
about it, God will discipline you. He will do it for your
good. However, I think this aspect of Christ's love for us is so
often misunderstood. In today's culture of "good vibes only,"
we run from the idea of accountability or discipline. This has
kept many from exploring the faith and even driven people
away. This misunderstanding is having serious implications.
We may also misunderstand God's discipline as the work of
the devil. That is, instead of letting the discipline of the Lord
mature and convict us, we blame the enemy.

TAKE HEART

Consider a time the Lord disciplined you. What did you learn?

TAKE ACTION

Make a list of areas where the Lord is working on you. What
is holding you back from receiving His loving correction?

REFRAIN

Now no discipline seems to be joyful at the time, but grievous. Yet afterward it yields the peaceful fruit of righteousness in those who have been trained by it.
—HEBREWS 12:11, MEV

W E ALL PROBABLY know we should not eat a lot of sugar. There are countless health consequences from having too much sugar all the time—everything from diabetes to obesity to increased risk of cancer. We are called to steward our health. Yes, God gave us amazing foods to eat, and moderation is critical. But we do ourselves much good by limiting sugar.

TAKE HEART

Are you a sugar addict? What areas do you struggle with nutritionally?

TAKE ACTION

Fast for twenty-four hours. Drink only water. Journal how you feel during that time.

Day 322
A CONSUMING FIRE

Therefore, since we are receiving a kingdom that cannot be shaken, let us be thankful, and so worship God acceptably with reverence and awe, for our "God is a consuming fire."
—HEBREW 12:28–29

JESUS IS AMAZING. Yes, He is tender, loving, mighty, forgiving, and filled with grace and mercy...but He is also a consuming fire! Not a candle. Not a flashlight. *Fire.*

Sometimes we unintentionally put God in a box. We kind of downplay His power and majesty. We forget just how powerful He is. We get so many images of Jesus sitting in a boat or walking with the disciples that we don't think about His mighty power.

Lord, let us worship You in awe and reverence. You are a consuming fire, not a fireplace. You desire our entire hearts.

TAKE HEART

Are you using God like a bonfire to stay warm and roast marshmallows, or are you jumping into His consuming fire?

TAKE ACTION

Reflect, and be honest with God and yourself. What is the most common perspective you have of God, Jesus, and the Holy Spirit? Is it power and fire? Remember, He is a mighty God.

ENTERTAINING ANGELS

Do not forget to show hospitality to strangers, for by so doing some people have shown hospitality to angels without knowing it.
—HEBREWS 13:2

EVEN IN THIS hyperconnected world with all its technology, phones, and computers, we have what has been called an "epidemic of loneliness." As a matter of fact, research has shown that the *more* you are on social media, the *lonelier* you feel. What a sad irony.

God is a God of relationship. That is one of the game-changing realities of a personal relationship with Jesus Christ. But Christ is also adamant about us being in relationship with each other. In this scripture He tells us to entertain strangers. When we do, we are actually at times entertaining angels. How incredible is it to think you have been with angels?

TAKE HEART

How do you feel around strangers? Nervous? Scared? Anxious? Excited? Why?

TAKE ACTION

Strike up a conversation with a stranger. Challenge yourself. You never know, he or she just might be an angel.

Day 324
COUNT IT PURE JOY

*Consider it pure joy, my brothers and sisters, whenever you face
trials of many kinds, because you know that the testing of your
faith produces perseverance. Let perseverance finish its work so
that you may be mature and complete, not lacking anything.*
—JAMES 1:2–4

D O YOU KNOW people who tend to deal poorly with
struggle? Some can be easily hurt and cannot handle too
much. They don't like to be uncomfortable and don't do well
in the heat of trouble. The problem is, avoiding struggle at all
costs actually makes things worse in the long run.

Here James explains how important it is to have trials in
our lives. He says we are to count them all joy. He tells us
that it builds perseverance, which helps us become "mature
and complete," lacking nothing. Did you catch this wisdom
coming from Jesus' half-brother? We would be wise to heed
these words.

TAKE HEART

How do you tend to respond to struggle and trial?

TAKE ACTION

Think about a trial or a struggle you are having right now.
Are you counting it all joy?

Day 325
BE WISE!

If any of you lacks wisdom, let him ask of God, who gives to all men liberally and without criticism, and it will be given to him.
—JAMES 1:5, MEV

SOMETIMES THE THINGS we need to do are super practical. Yes, God can do anything, anytime, any way. However, we can use wisdom to make better decisions. Eating good, healthy fats is a great way to improve your health and wellness. Good sources of fat include olive oil, avocado, flaxseed, nuts and seeds, raw butter and cheese, grass-fed beef and dairy, free-range chicken and eggs, and wild-caught fish, particularly salmon. These are some of best sources of energy, are essential for cell wall integrity, help the body burn fat and balance hormones, are anti-inflammatory, and aid in the transport of vitamins (namely A, D, E, and K).[1] The benefits of good fats are abundant. In fact, I have had patients heal from depression from just changing their diets!

TAKE HEART

Look at the list of good fats. How are you doing? Are you eating good fats?

TAKE ACTION

Go shopping (or throw out the junk). Stock your pantry with good choices.

GOD WILL NEVER TEMPT YOU

*When tempted, no one should say, "God is tempting
me." For God cannot be tempted by evil, nor does he
tempt anyone; but each person is tempted when they are
dragged away by their own evil desire and enticed.*
—JAMES 1:13–14

HAVE YOU EVER said "God is tempting me"? Over the years we all may have said or thought something like this. However, Jesus warns us that He will never tempt us. Only the devil does that. God does only good. He may allow the devil to tempt us, but only for our benefit—to help us refine our faith and to grow and mature. It is critical we keep this understanding and perspective, or we will often blame God for sins we choose to do. The devil is real. The devil tempts us. But the Lord allows us, through Him, to overcome all sin.

TAKE HEART

Do you blame God and think He is tempting you? Does this scripture give you a different perspective?

TAKE ACTION

Take responsibility for your sinful actions.

ARE YOU DECEIVING YOURSELF?

*Do not merely listen to the word, and so
deceive yourselves. Do what it says.*
—JAMES 1:22

REMEMBER THE SAYING "Ignorance is bliss"? Maybe you have met people who prefer to keep their heads in the sand because then they do not need to change anything or think critically. I see this often in relation to people's health. They just want to remain ignorant instead of learning and making changes to their lifestyle choices. But here is the reality: ignorance isn't bliss—it is deadly.

This is what James is trying to get us to see here. Don't just be a hearer of the Word; do something. Be a doer of the Word. He is saying, "Don't deceive yourselves by only listening." Think of it like this: if I sat and listened to a person talk about exercise but didn't actually do any exercise, I would just be deceiving myself. But the stakes are much higher with our faith.

TAKE HEART

Are you a hearer or a doer?

TAKE ACTION

What areas of your life and faith do you need to be a *doer* in?

EVEN THE DEMONS BELIEVE THAT

In the same way, faith by itself, if it is not accompanied by action, is dead. But someone will say, "You have faith; I have deeds." Show me your faith without deeds, and I will show you my faith by my deeds. You believe that there is one God. Good! Even the demons believe that—and shudder.
—JAMES 2:17–19

THE BOOK OF James is very challenging. It is a kick in the butt. A reminder that our lives should bear fruit. A reminder that if we truly have faith, that if we truly believe and are saved by Jesus, we should have a life filled with good works. James insists that just believing in God is not enough—even the devil does that! He also tells us that faith without good works is dead. Dead. Remember, folks, Jesus' brother is writing this.

If we have been saved by Jesus, our lives need to show the evidence. That evidence includes works in our transformed lives.

TAKE HEART

Do you struggle with this? Does this sound like works-based theology? What does this passage mean to you?

TAKE ACTION

Is your faith dead? Can people look at your life and see fruit? Faith should create action. Put action to your faith today.

Day 329
CAN A FIG TREE BEAR OLIVES?

*With the tongue we praise our Lord and Father, and with it
we curse human beings, who have been made in God's likeness. Out of the same mouth come praise and cursing. My
brothers and sisters, this should not be. Can both fresh water
and salt water flow from the same spring? My brothers
and sisters, can a fig tree bear olives, or a grapevine bear
figs? Neither can a salt spring produce fresh water.*
—JAMES 3:9–12

JAMES CONTINUES HIS strong admonishment about how we speak. He gives strong warnings about the power of the tongue to destroy and also to reveal our hearts. Your words are an overflow of your heart. We can learn a lot about ourselves and others by the words that come out of our mouths.

Words matter. How we speak to ourselves and each other matters. A lot. We have all experienced the truth that the power of life and death resides in the tongue. We can all look back and remember words that were spoken to us—whether edifying or hurtful. How you speak about your health also matters. How you speak about others' health matters. Be careful; words have power. Speak life.

TAKE HEART

Do you speak life or death?

TAKE ACTION

Today, be extra aware of the words coming out of your mouth and the words you speak to yourself.

WISDOM?

*Who is wise and understanding among you? Let them show it
by their good life, by deeds done in the humility that comes
from wisdom. But if you harbor bitter envy and selfish ambition in your hearts, do not boast about it or deny the truth.
Such "wisdom" does not come down from heaven but is earthly,
unspiritual, demonic. For where you have envy and selfish
ambition, there you find disorder and every evil practice.*
—JAMES 3:13–16

Wow, James is a stiff cup of truth coffee. What timely, relevant, and straight-shooting teaching he has for us. Your
life should be filled with good deeds done with humility, not
worldly, fleshly wisdom. When we have envy, selfish ambition,
and boasting in our hearts, that is not from heaven but from
the devil. And it never works in the long run. You can find endless fleshly wisdom in any bookstore or on YouTube or Facebook. This is what James warns us about. Don't fall for it; it is
literally the work of the devil. If we desire wisdom from God,
we must know Him, His ways, and His Word.

TAKE HEART

What kind of wisdom do you seek? What kind of wisdom do
you share?

TAKE ACTION

God has a lot of practical advice. Reflect on your heart. Are
you too focused on this world's "wisdom"? What do you think
Jesus would say?

Day 331
SUBMIT YOURSELVES TO GOD

Submit yourselves, then, to God. Resist the devil, and he will flee from you. Come near to God and he will come near to you. Wash your hands, you sinners, and purify your hearts, you double-minded. Grieve, mourn and wail. Change your laughter to mourning and your joy to gloom.
—JAMES 4:7–9

HAVE YOU OVERCOMPLICATED your life? Are you burning the candle at both ends? Living a fast-food, caffeine-fueled, stressed-out, sleep-deprived life? Oftentimes when we are not feeling or hearing well physically, emotionally, and spiritually, the problem is *us*—the choices we are making. James gives us some profound advice here: (1) submit to God (not the world), (2) resist the devil, and (3) don't be double-minded.

This is so simple but life changing. I often tell patients to not let the simplicity of the health recommendations make them seem unimportant. Breathing is pretty simple. But don't do it for a few minutes and you will find out how important it is. Christ told us the simple will confound the wise.

TAKE HEART

Where have you overcomplicated or overwhelmed your life? What needs to go?

TAKE ACTION

Prune the vine. List two to three days' worth of your typical schedule and everything you do. Review, reflect, and pray. Where are you double-minded?

YOUR LIFE IS A MIST

*Now listen, you who say, "Today or tomorrow we will go to
this or that city, spend a year there, carry on business and
make money." Why, you do not even know what will happen
tomorrow. What is your life? You are a mist that appears
for a little while and then vanishes. Instead, you ought to
say, "If it is the Lord's will, we will live and do this or that."*
—JAMES 4:13–15

WE WILL ALL die someday. We have no idea what
tomorrow will bring. We often make big plans after
going to a seminar, but Jesus has some advice for us. He
reminds us that our lives are like a mist that appears for a
minute and then is gone.

Your life is a mist. Don't waste it on things that don't matter.
Don't waste it on things that will rot and waste away. Don't
stress out about tomorrow, and don't boast or brag about all
your big goals or plans. Your life is a mist. A vapor. Then it
is gone.

TAKE HEART

Have you let the stress and worry about tomorrow affect your
life today?

TAKE ACTION

Just for today, stay in the moment. Focus on today; it may be
all we have.

SIN OF OMISSION

*If anyone, then, knows the good they ought to
do and doesn't do it, it is sin for them.*
—JAMES 4:17

IN HEALTH CARE doctors can commit malpractice by doing something they shouldn't have (such as removing a wrong organ) or *not* doing something they should have (such as missing a test result). Here James shows us how this idea relates to our relationship with God. He tells us it is a sin to know the right thing to do and not do it.

This takes righteous living to a whole different level. I think we often look at *doing good* like we deserve a pat on the back, as if it is something extra, like we deserve extra credit from Jesus. But we rarely consider it a sin to *not* do something. It is the sin of omission.

TAKE HEART

How many times have we felt the nudge from God to do the right thing but not done it?

TAKE ACTION

Take action today. Do the right thing. Living a godly life is about not only steering clear of things you can't do but also doing the godly works you can.

Day 334
A WARNING AGAINST
SELF-INDULGING

*You have lived on earth in luxury and self-indulgence. You
have fattened yourselves in the day of slaughter.*
—JAMES 5:5

WE HAVE ALL read or heard the stories or warnings about
how difficult it is for the rich to come into the kingdom
of heaven. We have heard the warnings about how money can
become an idol in our lives and how the love of it is the root
of all evil. We often read these scriptures and say, "Well, I
am not that rich." The purpose of today's devotional is not
to debate whether you are rich or not; it is to consider how
focused we are on *self*.

Here James calls us out on our self-indulgent lifestyles. You
don't have to be rich to live a self-focused life. Especially in
America, our lives are often full of indulgences and comfort.
We believe bigger is better. We overeat, overspend, oversleep,
overstimulate, and overmedicate. James is trying to warn us:
this is not what the Lord desires for us.

TAKE HEART

Would you consider yourself a person who overindulges? Do
you eat too much? Spend too much?

TAKE ACTION

List one or two areas where you need restraint. Take these to
God, and find ways to be held accountable.

Day 335
JUST A LITTLE PATIENCE

Brothers and sisters, as an example of patience in the
face of suffering, take the prophets who spoke in the
name of the Lord. As you know, we count as blessed
those who have persevered. You have heard of Job's per-
severance and have seen what the Lord finally brought
about. The Lord is full of compassion and mercy.
—JAMES 5:10–11

As we have noted before, we live in a quick-fix society. We want everything yesterday. If we have pain, we want a pill. If we need to lose weight, we want a surgery. Such an ungodly perspective has sent us down a road that leads to destruction. It has created a culture that leads to divorce and increased anxiety and suicide.

Here James implores us to value patience. He reminds us how crucial it is for us to persevere. He uses the powerful example of Job. In fact, we often use the phrase *the patience of Job* when describing a person with supernatural patience. Too often we are missing the blessings and plans the Lord has for us because we are not exercising patience and perseverance.

TAKE HEART

Do you struggle with patience? What is a time or an area of your life where you quit before you should have?

TAKE ACTION

Reflect on a time where you persevered. Think about what would have happened if you hadn't.

Day 336
ANOINT THEM WITH OIL

*Is anyone among you sick? Let them call the elders of the church
to pray over them and anoint them with oil in the name of the
Lord. And the prayer offered in faith will make the sick person
well; the Lord will raise them up....Therefore confess your sins to
each other and pray for each other so that you may be healed.
The prayer of a righteous person is powerful and effective.*
—JAMES 5:14–16

OVER THE YEARS many have told me they "have tried every-thing" to get better. But this is often not the case. They usually mean they did whatever the doctor told them to do.

James lays out clear instruction for those who are sick: call on the elders of the church to anoint the sick person with oil in the Lord's name, and then pray. Prayer offered in faith will make the sick person well. Praise the Lord!

Why do we do this so rarely? We find it less weird to go under anesthesia for surgery than to be prayed over and anointed with oil. Think of how many people—including you—could be healed by being willing to take this step of faith and obedience. Have you really tried everything?

TAKE HEART

Have you ever been prayed for and anointed with oil? Are you willing to be?

TAKE ACTION

If you or someone you know is sick, find a person or a church willing to pray and anoint with oil.

DESIGNED TO HEAL

Day 337

REFINED BY FIRE

These have come so that the proven genuineness of your faith—of greater worth than gold, which perishes even though refined by fire—may result in praise, glory and honor when Jesus Christ is revealed.
—1 Peter 1:7

WE ALMOST ALWAYS perceive things we don't like as "bad." When we go through trials and struggles, we say these are "bad times." We all go through intense moments, but Peter encourages us to reframe these crucible moments as like a refiner's fire. It's what proves whether we are genuine. And it *results in praise, glory, and honor* when Jesus Christ is revealed.

What a perspective shift. The trials lead to glory. The pain has a purpose. The refiner's fire is critical to revealing who and whose you truly are.

We often do anything we can to avoid struggle, and as a result, we have become a largely soft, selfish culture. You don't build muscle without stressing it. You don't birth a child without some birth pains. It's crucial we reframe struggle and see God working in it.

TAKE HEART

How do you respond during trials and fire? What's a better perspective?

TAKE ACTION

Stop avoiding hard things. It's critical to stay in the fight. It's worth it!

BE HOLY BECAUSE I AM HOLY

Therefore, with minds that are alert and fully sober, set your hope on the grace to be brought to you when Jesus Christ is revealed at his coming. As obedient children, do not con-form to the evil desires you had when you lived in igno-rance. But just as he who called you is holy, so be holy in all you do; for it is written: "Be holy, because I am holy."
—1 PETER 1:13–16

THE BIBLE IS amazing. The truth about life, death, healing, hope, purpose, and so much more is found in these pages. So many (even all) of the problems people face in this world are addressed directly in the living pages of the Bible— including this passage. If we simply followed this truth, we would be transformed and so would the world: (1) prepare your mind for action; (2) be self-controlled; (3) set your hope fully on the grace given from Christ; (4) do not conform to evil desire; and (5) be holy because He is holy. I believe many of us simply don't even try to be holy. We have believed the devil's lies. But we can live holy lives through Christ and the power of the Holy Spirit.

TAKE HEART

When you reflect on this scripture, how are you doing? Do you strive to live a holy life?

TAKE ACTION

"Be holy in all you do."

TASTE AND SEE THAT THE LORD IS GOOD

Therefore, rid yourselves of all malice and all deceit, hypocrisy, envy, and slander of every kind. Like newborn babies, crave pure spiritual milk, so that by it you may grow up in your salvation, now that you have tasted that the Lord is good.
—1 PETER 2:1–3

"CRAVE PURE SPIRITUAL milk"! Working in health care, I'm often asked, "What should I eat?" or "What vitamin do I need?" Now these are, of course, good and reasonable questions, but they are never a substitute for spiritual milk—the living Word of God, prayer, and direct communication with your heavenly Father. We are called to *crave* the spiritual milk. Do you crave it? Have you ever tasted it? Does this seem weird or odd to you?

Because we have partaken of it so often, we often crave the world, the ways of sin. Here we are encouraged to taste of the good Father. Drink of Him, and never grow thirsty or weary.

TAKE HEART

Have you tasted the goodness of God? Do you *crave Him*? What would that look like?

TAKE ACTION

Take a moment right now to pray that the Lord will give you a taste for Him—for His glory and goodness—and that you will crave Him.

ABSTAIN FROM THE PASSIONS OF THE FLESH

Dear friends, I urge you, as foreigners and exiles, to abstain from sinful desires, which wage war against your soul.
—1 PETER 2:11

SOME POPULAR SAYINGS nowadays are "Follow your bliss" or "Choose your dream," etc. Now I'm not saying these are all bad, but I will tell you that my flesh (sinful nature) often leads me down a messy path. We are really good at fooling ourselves. Peter warns us to abstain from passions of the flesh because they wage war against our souls. That sounds like a very stern warning!

We want to follow Jesus and His plans, not our plans. Remember the old bracelets with "WWJD" on them? What would Jesus do? That's always a good question.

TAKE HEART

Whom are you following: your flesh or Jesus?

TAKE ACTION

What area do you need to put the brakes on? What is waging war against your soul?

Day 341
ZEALOUS FOR GOD

Who is going to harm you if you are eager to do good? But
even if you should suffer for what is right, you are blessed....
Always be prepared to give an answer to everyone who asks
you to give the reason for the hope that you have. But do this
with gentleness and respect, keeping a clear conscience, so
that those who speak maliciously against your good behavior
in Christ may be ashamed of their slander. For it is better, if
it is God's will, to suffer for doing good than for doing evil.
—1 PETER 3:13–17

MOTHER TERESA IS credited with saying, "If you hold an anti-war rally, I shall not attend. But if you hold a pro-peace rally, invite me."[1] She chose to focus on peace, not war. We have only a limited time each day. We can spend it fighting evil (there is a time and place for that) or glorifying God by being zealous for Him.

Most struggles in our lives are not from the devil but from our personal choices. Time after time, we are encouraged to choose holy living. We are promised it is possible. We have seen examples. God assures us that even if we suffer while doing good, we're blessed! So we can't really lose! Go do some good.

TAKE HEART

Are you busy doing good?

TAKE ACTION

Today, stop blaming circumstance, God, or the devil. Take responsibility for your actions. *Do good.*

YOUR BODY IS A GIFT

As everyone has received a gift, even so serve one another
with it, as good stewards of the manifold grace of God.
—1 PETER 4:10, MEV

SUPPOSE YOU HAD a pet cat that you fed only potato chips and soda and he sat around all day. What do you think would happen? Would the cat get sick? Why? Now take the cat out of the scenario and insert yourself. We are not designed to eat these foods. Then we wonder why we are getting sicker. Remember, your body is a gift from God. Treat it well, as a good steward.

TAKE HEART

Why do we often take better care of our cars and animals than we do the bodies God gave us?

TAKE ACTION

Review how you feed your animals or maintain your car. Ask yourself whether you are stewarding those things better than your divine design.

Day 343
CAST ALL YOUR ANXIETY ON HIM

Cast all your anxiety on him because he cares for you.
—1 PETER 5:7

ONE OF THE biggest, most common health concerns of men, women, and children is anxiety. Almost every year, the rate of it goes up. More people than ever are attempting to cope with anxiety through medications, distractions, alcohol, or illegal or legal drugs. We are almost to the point where anxiety is accepted as normal. Yet as usual God knows our struggles. He spoke very directly to anxiety.

Think about this: the scripture holds the answer to one of today's most common diagnoses. *"Cast all your anxiety on him because he cares for you."* How incredible that we have a caring Father who is the Great Physician, our healer and provider—Jehovah Rapha and Jehovah Jireh. We can take it all to Him. Psalm 55:22 says it this way: "Cast your cares on the LORD and he will sustain you."

TAKE HEART

Do you struggle with anxiety? Do you cast it on the Lord?

TAKE ACTION

Imagine Jesus walking into the room, face to face with you, during a time you were experiencing anxiety. What do you think He would say?

Day 344

SLOW DOWN

Cast all your care upon Him, because He cares for you.
—1 Peter 5:7, mev

In 2008, Dr. Robert Leahy stated, "The average high school kid today has the same level of anxiety as the average psychiatric patient in the early 1950s."[1] Consider this for a moment. Also consider that as a society we take more medications for anxiety and depression and mental health than we ever have—yet we are sicker and struggling in these areas more than ever.

We saw major disruptions during the pandemic, of course, but it runs deeper than that. The speed of today's world is out of alignment with God's design! We are not designed for this pace. No pill will fix it.

TAKE HEART

Are you getting sucked into today's pace? Burning the candle at both ends? Living on adrenaline and coffee and less sleep? How is it working?

TAKE ACTION

Disconnect to reconnect. Look at your life and areas you can unplug from the ways of the world. You won't regret it.

Day 345

EVERYTHING YOU NEED

*His divine power has given us everything we need for a
godly life through our knowledge of him who called us by
his own glory and goodness. Through these he has given us
his very great and precious promises, so that through them
you may participate in the divine nature, having escaped
the corruption in the world caused by evil desires.*
—2 PETER 1:3–4

HAVE YOU EVER thought or said, "It's too hard"—maybe
in reference to some aspect of your walk with Christ or
to taking care of yourself? Peter talks directly to this kind of
thinking and lets us know that no excuse holds up. God's divine
power has given us everything we need for life and godliness.

This is really important. Whenever you think that you
can't do something, that it's too hard or is impossible, you
must remind yourself that God has given you everything you
need for life and godliness. *Everything.* So many times we
complain about what we don't have or make excuses, but God
says we have *everything* we need. Praise the Lord! Let this
encourage you.

TAKE HEART

Is this your perspective? Or do you find yourself talking and
thinking about what you think you don't have?

TAKE ACTION

Today every time you think you need something, remind
yourself of this scripture.

BEWARE OF COUNTERFEITS

But there were also false prophets among the people, just as there will be false teachers among you. They will secretly introduce destructive heresies, even denying the sovereign Lord who bought them—bringing swift destruction on themselves.
—2 PETER 2:1

IN THEIR RESEARCH, authors Eric Schlosser and Charles Wilson found that the typical major fast-food chain's "strawberry milkshake" recipe contains a whole paragraph's worth of chemicals—but *no* strawberries![1] It is a chemical concoction that *tastes* like a strawberry milkshake, but it is not! It is an illusion. It's like a candle that smells like pumpkin pie, but you are not designed to eat it. We need to be our own advocates as we navigate our food choices and feed our bodies, which are gifts from God.

TAKE HEART

Do you read labels? Do you know how to identify some of the *worst* ingredients for your health?

TAKE ACTION

Next time you go shopping, try not to buy anything that you cannot pronounce all the ingredients of.

A MAN IS A SLAVE TO WHATEVER HAS MASTERED HIM

They promise them freedom, while they them-
selves are slaves of depravity—for "people are
slaves to whatever has mastered them."
—2 PETER 2:19

WE ARE ALL "slaves" to something. We are slaves to Christ or slaves to sin. We are slaves to whatever has mastered us. Has Jesus mastered you? Is He your everything? Or does the world have your heart? Have you been mastered by sin, lust, greed, flesh, porn, work, sex, addiction, or anger instead of Jesus?

Many of us, especially those who were saved later in life, had built a life of sinful habits. We were slaves to sin—maybe not even knowing it was sin. Now we are learning and surrendering and being molded by the Potter. *Thank You, Jesus, for being a wonderful and loving master.*

TAKE HEART

Do you have areas of your heart or lifestyle where you are still mastered by sin?

TAKE ACTION

Take action. Take your needs to the Lord. Surrender. Let Him be your master.

Day 348
NOTHING BUT THE BLOOD OF JESUS

*But if we walk in the light as He is in the light, we
have fellowship one with another, and the blood
of Jesus Christ His Son cleanses us from all sin.*
—1 JOHN 1:7, MEV

THE BIBLE TALKS a lot about the blood, making countless
references to blood and its importance. We know that
ingesting large amounts of processed food and sugar has a
negative impact on our blood and is linked to increases in
diabetes. This is a good example of how we can mess up our
blood by the choices we make. The way we care for ourselves
has consequences. We reap what we sow—cause and effect.
Our choices matter, and they affect us at the cellular level.
The way we eat, move, and think affects our blood.

TAKE HEART

When you are eating, do you ever think about what this is
doing to your cells? Is it making your blood healthier?

TAKE ACTION

Say a prayer right now about your blood. Ask the Lord to
restore your blood and cover you in the blood of Jesus.

THE MAN WHO DOES THE WILL OF GOD LIVES FOREVER

Do not love the world or anything in the world. If anyone loves the world, love for the Father is not in them. For everything in the world—the lust of the flesh, the lust of the eyes, and the pride of life—comes not from the Father but from the world. The world and its desires pass away, but whoever does the will of God lives forever.
—1 JOHN 2:15-17

A s you have worked through these scriptures, I pray you have noticed how much effort the Bible makes to remind us to not love this world or get sucked into materialism, greed, and fleshly desires. Numerous scriptures are dedicated to this important perspective. We should make sure we are heeding this advice. John tells us here to not love *anything* in the world. If we do love the world, the love of the *Father* is not in us. As we are marketed to, as the world has more and more access to our hearts through social media, television, etc., we must be intentional and careful to not let our hearts be corrupted. The stakes are high. The call is real. This is not a guess or a suggestion.

TAKE HEART

Are there areas of this world that are idols to you?

TAKE ACTION

Where does the world have some of your heart? Reflect on these areas. When did this start? Do you want to break the chains?

CHILDREN OF GOD SHOULD NOT BE THIS SICK!

*Beloved, now are we children of God, and it has not
yet been revealed what we shall be. But we know
that when He appears, we shall be like Him.*
—1 JOHN 3:2, MEV

HERE IS AN unbelievable, heartbreaking statistic: About 43 percent of our children are diagnosed with a chronic health condition, rising to 54 percent when obesity and other risks are factored in.[1] This is up from 31 percent in 1988.[2] And about 20 percent of children are diagnosed with a neurological disease.[3] Most of these diseases are considered something they will have the rest of their lives.

As believers, we know God designed us intricately, in His likeness and image. The cause of this disease problem is not God; it is *us*—our choices and lifestyles. *Lord, have mercy and help us turn this ship around for our dear children.*

TAKE HEART

What do you think about this statistic? Why have our kids become so sick?

TAKE ACTION

Some are warning that this generation of kids may die at a younger age than their parents.[4] What a sickening possibility. We must look at what we are feeding, injecting, and surrounding our children with. Are you helping your kids thrive?

Day 351

GOD LOVES HIS CHILDREN

See what great love the Father has lavished on us, that we should be called children of God! And that is what we are! The reason the world does not know us is that it did not know him.
—1 JOHN 3:1

OFTENTIMES WHEN WE read the Holy Scriptures, we can feel the heart of the Father. As a parent, I think it's almost impossible to miss how the Lord talks to us. He loves us; we are His children. He lavishes love on us, and at the same time He needs to correct us, mold us, disciple us. Sometimes we can get stuck or focused on only one aspect of God. This is OK, as we may need to dive deep in different seasons. But it is also important *we never forget His love for us.*

If you are a parent, you will understand this love at some level. Even when your kids are driving you crazy, your heart is filled with love for them. God is like this, but He is perfect. Be in awe of being a child of God.

TAKE HEART

Do you feel like a child of God? Is that your perspective? Or do you often feel like you're in trouble, guilty, or shamed?

TAKE ACTION

Reflect on your upbringing or maybe how you now parent. Has this affected your perspective of being a child of God?

WHAT DO YOU CONFESS?

Every spirit that confesses that Jesus Christ has come in the
flesh is from God, and every spirit that does not confess
that Jesus Christ has come in the flesh is not from God.
—1 JOHN 4:2–3, MEV

DR. RICHARD CABOT of Harvard Medical School once said, "The wisdom of the body is responsible for 90% of the hope of the patients to recover. The body has a super wisdom that is in favor of life, rather than death. This is the power that we depend on for life. All doctors are responsible for letting their patients know of this great force working within them."[1] This is a great reminder. The only thing I would say is that it is not 90 percent; it is 100 percent the power of God. Wouldn't it be great if our health-care system had this mindset? Instead, we often think the opposite: 90 percent man and 10 percent God.

TAKE HEART

How do you view healing? Is it from God? From man?

TAKE ACTION

Challenge some of your assumptions or beliefs about current health care. Are you having more faith and giving more credit to man than the One who *created* man?

GREATER IS HE THAT IS IN YOU

*You, dear children, are from God and have over-
come them, because the one who is in you is
greater than the one who is in the world.*
—1 JOHN 4:4

IT ALWAYS BREAKS my heart when I meet a defeated, "woe
is me" Christian. I know that we have ups and downs and
that life circumstances can at times overwhelm us, but the
truth is that we have God. We have Jesus. We have the Holy
Spirit. Greater is He who is in you! If our lives are only as
good as our circumstances, we are in trouble. Just ask Paul,
John, John the Baptist, Job, and countless others. We are
always "good" because our God is good. This is one of the
defining attributes of a Christian—a never-ending, bottom-
less, overflowing sense of hope. Not hope in ourselves or circumstances but *hope in God*!

TAKE HEART

Do you feel this hope? Be honest: Do you spend more of your
day feeling bitter or sad? What do you think Jesus would say
about that?

TAKE ACTION

Meditate on this scripture. Let it soothe your heart, your fears,
your anxieties, your grumblings. Let it heal and restore you!

Day 354
LOVE

Let us love one another, for love comes from God....God is love....
We love because he first loved us....For whoever does not love
their brother and sister, whom they have seen, cannot love God,
whom they have not seen. And he has given us this command:
Anyone who loves God must also love their brother and sister.
—1 John 4:7–8, 19–21

I BELIEVE THIS MAY be a day that will change your life. In fact, I encourage you to read 1 John 4:7–21 in its entirety. God's love for you and your love for others are interconnected. This allows you to reflect on your own heart and be caught up in the wonder of God's love. His love is given first to you, and out of that love—and only out of that love—can you truly love others. If you are like me and many others, you have family drama. We all have people in our lives that we struggle to love. It's critical, as this passage shows, to allow God to show you a way to love them. It may seem impossible, but we know through Christ all things are possible. This one is holding so many believers back. Let this passage heal your heart for others.

TAKE HEART

Are there people in your life that you hate or dislike?

TAKE ACTION

Take those people to God. Begin praying daily for them. Watch the miracle happen in your heart.

HIS COMMANDS ARE
NOT BURDENSOME

This is love for God: to keep his commands. And his com-
mands are not burdensome, for everyone born of God over-
comes the world. This is the victory that has overcome the
world, even our faith. Who is it that overcomes the world?
Only the one who believes that Jesus is the Son of God.
—1 JOHN 5:3–5

WHEN WE HEAR things like "Follow my commands," we tend to think they indicate tyranny or dictatorship. Our natural response is often negative. But consider this: if you were lost in the woods but had a cell phone, and on the other end of the line was a knowledgeable person who was going to help you get to safety, how would you feel about the commands that person gave you? You would probably feel pretty thankful. This is the posture we are to take toward our all-knowing God and His Word. We are not to be burdened by His commands, as they give us life.

TAKE HEART

How do you feel about God's Word? His commands?

TAKE ACTION

Reframe. Consider the Old Testament. The Israelites praised God for His laws. They knew they were chosen by God to receive His guidance. Is that how you feel?

BELIEVE

Who is it that overcomes the world, but the one
who believes that Jesus is the Son of God?
—1 JOHN 5:5, MEV

THE ENEMY LIKES to confuse us. With contradictory science, constantly changing moral standards, cancel culture, fad diets, and so many opinions out there, it is easy for us to get distracted. Whom do we want to believe: God or mankind? This may not be a popular message, but that does not make it untrue. Jesus spoke perfect truth, and He was hung on a cross.

TAKE HEART

Are there areas you are afraid to make a stand for Christ in? Are there areas where the world has confused you or infiltrated your mind and heart?

TAKE ACTION

The only way to combat confusion is with truth. God's Word is truth. Dive in daily.

Day 357
FACE TO FACE

I have much to write to you, but I do not want to use
paper and ink. Instead, I hope to visit you and talk with
you face to face, so that our joy may be complete.
—2 JOHN 12

IN THESE TIMES of technological advance, online meet-ings, text messages, Snapchat, and more, it has become very rare to actually meet face to face. Even back in the "old days" people knew there was something special about being together, breaking bread, shaking hands, hugging. Have you found yourself isolated? Lonely? Even in the midst of our most "connected" time, our kids are considered the loneliest generation in history.

If you're feeling lonely or isolated, get out and be with others—especially other believers, such as at church. Don't be socially distanced. Don't be afraid to be with others and even to hug them. It mattered back in John's time, and it matters today.

TAKE HEART

Do you enjoy being with others? Why or why not? Did Jesus?

TAKE ACTION

Host a get together. Invite some people to dinner. Join a small group. Volunteer.

Day 358
WALKING IN TRUTH

Dear friend, I pray that you may enjoy good health and that all may go well with you, even as your soul is getting along well. It gave me great joy when some believers came and testified about your faithfulness to the truth, telling how you continue to walk in it. I have no greater joy than to hear that my children are walking in the truth.
—3 John 2–4

I LOVE THIS VISUAL: walking in truth. It demonstrates action, movement, going forward. If you know the truth but you're not walking in it, does it really matter? The devil knows the truth, but he is not walking in the truth. Some scriptures we have discussed even say that if we know the right thing to do and we don't, that is a sin. John says he has no greater joy than hearing that people are walking in the truth. That means taking action—and taking kingdom territory in the name of Jesus. What an amazing reminder! I also love that it says "walk," not sprint. Remember, it is a journey, a marathon that is at a pace we can all do.

TAKE HEART

Are you moving? Are you taking faith-filled action? Is your faith being put into action?

TAKE ACTION

Make a move today. Walk it out. Let someone be touched by the Holy Spirit through you.

CONTEND FOR THE FAITH

*Dear friends, although I was very eager to write to
you about the salvation we share, I felt compelled
to write and urge you to contend for the faith that
was once for all entrusted to God's holy people.*
—JUDE 3

A s we have journeyed through the New Testament with
an eye and ear toward being well and whole, it is impossible to not feel the call to action—to engage, to contend for
the faith. The scriptures are definitely not shy about the fact
that as believers we will face struggles and burdens; things
won't seem fair.

Just look at the disciples and other early believers. It's not
a glamorous, prosperity-gospel life. Yet it is a life well lived, a
life worthy of the call. They contended for their faith and the
faith of others. They fought the good fight. They ran the race
daily.

TAKE HEART

Are you contending for your faith? Are you contending for
others' faith? What holds you back or trips you up?

TAKE ACTION

Get involved in the battle. Show up. We fight for things we
value and believe are important.

THE TIME IS NOW

*Blessed is he who reads and those who hear the
words of this prophecy and keep those things
which are written in it, for the time is near.*
—REVELATION 1:3, MEV

WE MUST REMEMBER how blessed we are to have the inspired Word of God to read and reference and hold dear to our hearts. Many who went before us did not have these inspired, God-breathed words. Let us cling to them as if they are our oxygen tank—because they are, even in our struggles. Remember, John wrote this while exiled to a remote island; he was not on vacation. We can find great hope in this Book.

TAKE HEART

Imagine being John, with everything you had seen, and then the Lord gives you this vision. How would you feel? Encouraged? Scared?

TAKE ACTION

We are reminded that the time is near. We are called to live a life of urgency. Are you?

Day 361

HOLY

"Holy, holy, holy, is the Lord God Almighty,"
who was, and is, and is to come.
—REVELATION 4:8

YES, JESUS IS our friend. Yes, we have a personal relationship with Him. However, make no mistake, when we come face to face with Him, we will fall on our faces.

He is holy. We would do well to remind ourselves of that truth. At times our comfort with His awesomeness can lead us to not take His ways very seriously. We are not God. We are not the judge. We are not the Alpha and Omega.

TAKE HEART

Do you ever get overwhelmed by the majesty of God? If it is not a regular occurrence, I suggest you let it become one. Our perspective of the majesty of God is critical to our worship of Him.

TAKE ACTION

Read Job 38. Be overwhelmed.

HINDSIGHT IS TWENTY-TWENTY

Nor did they repent of their murders, their magic arts
[pharmakeia], their sexual immorality, or their thefts.
—REVELATION 9:21

DO YOU REMEMBER being told to take a daily aspirin? Do you know that is no longer recommended for most healthy people? You may also be surprised to know the side effects from taking a daily aspirin, including increased risk of gastrointestinal bleeding.[1] Many of us have been conditioned to view medications like vitamins instead of chemicals that can be toxic. This erroneous view has had dramatic effects on our health. You would do yourself a huge favor by researching any pill or vaccine or chemical you put in, on, or around your body. You may be surprised.

TAKE HEART

God did not create you with a deficiency in prescription drugs. Focus on getting to the cause of the problem and not just medicating yourself.

TAKE ACTION

If you are taking any medications, whether prescription or over-the-counter, look them up online and read about the side effects.

Day 363
DRUGS DON'T HEAL—JESUS DOES

The light of a lamp shall shine in you no more, and the voice
of bridegroom and of bride shall be heard in you no more.
For your merchants were the great men of the earth, and
all nations were deceived by your sorcery [pharmakeia].
—REVELATION 18:23, MEV

THE UNITED STATES has about 4 percent of the world's population, yet we consume an estimated 75 percent of the world's prescription drugs.[1] When I share statistics like this one, people are often not surprised. It seems as though everyone knows we take a lot of medications and drugs in this country, and people just kind of shrug it off with "Well, what are we going to do?" or "Well, you know how Big Pharma is." I am always surprised they don't ask, "How is this working out?" It would be good news if it were paying off with good health. But that's not the case. The reality is we are getting *sicker*.

TAKE HEART

What do you think about all the medications people take? Do you think they are necessary? Do you think there are other ways to approach health than synthetic chemicals? Do you think disease is due to a lack of drugs?

TAKE ACTION

Review your and your family's lifestyles. Are you on medications? Do you have a desire or a conviction to get to the cause of your health problems instead of masking them with medications and drugs?

THE RIDER ON THE WHITE HORSE

I saw heaven opened. And there was a white horse. He who sat on it is called Faithful and True, and in righteousness He judges and wages war. His eyes are like a flame of fire, and on His head are many crowns. He has a name written, that no one knows but He Himself. He is clothed with a robe dipped in blood. His name is called The Word of God....Out of His mouth proceeds a sharp sword, with which He may strike the nations. "He shall rule them with an iron scepter."...On His robe and on His thigh He has a name written: King of kings and Lord of lords.
—REVELATION 19:11–16, MEV

JESUS DOES NOT mess around. He is the Lion and the Lamb. Unfortunately, at times we put Jesus in a little box, seeing Him as a guy walking around giving everyone hugs and handshakes like a politician. He is the King of kings. Today's passage should put fear and excitement in our hearts. This is critical to remember, as He resides within us, filling us with His power—resurrection power! All things are possible through Christ who gives us strength.

TAKE HEART

How does this Scripture passage make you feel? Imagine His return. This is our God!

TAKE ACTION

Does your perspective of God and His power reflect this description? How mighty is the God you serve? Do you talk and pray to Him like that?

Day 365

WATER OF LIFE

The Spirit and the bride say, "Come." Let him who hears say, "Come." Let him who is thirsty come. Let him who desires take the water of life freely.
—REVELATION 22:17, MEV

THESE ARE NEARLY the last words of the Holy Scriptures. They are Jesus' words to the world. A final call. An opportunity to drink the living water, to taste of His goodness forever. While we have talked a lot about caring for the bodies God has given us, make no mistake, we will all face the throne of judgment. Don't miss your chance. Don't settle for the things of this world. Call on the Lord. He will answer.

TAKE HEART

His desires are for you to drink of His goodness, to be saved. Seek Him. Yearn for Him.

TAKE ACTION

If you have any doubt about your salvation or relationship with the living Christ, pray to Him now. Ask Him to save you. Repent and be saved. Only He saves. Forever and ever. Amen.

NERVOUS SYSTEM

PARASYMPATHETIC

SYMPATHETIC

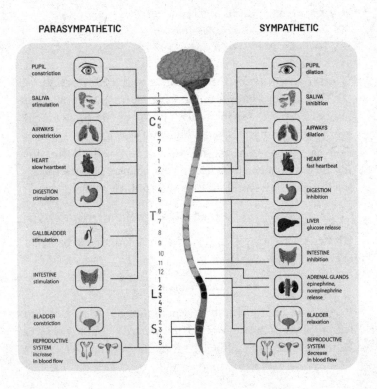

PUPIL
constriction

SALIVA
stimulation

AIRWAYS
constriction

HEART
slow heartbeat

DIGESTION
stimulation

GALLBLADDER
stimulation

INTESTINE
stimulation

BLADDER
constriction

REPRODUCTIVE
SYSTEM
increase
in blood flow

PUPIL
dilation

SALIVA
inhibition

AIRWAYS
dilation

HEART
fast heartbeat

DIGESTION
inhibition

LIVER
glucose release

INTESTINE
inhibition

ADRENAL GLANDS
epinephrine,
norepinephrine
release

BLADDER
relaxation

REPRODUCTIVE
SYSTEM
decrease
in blood flow

NOTES

Day 3

1. Tim Jewell, "How Long Does It Take for Sperm to Regenerate?
   What to Expect," Healthline, September 19, 2018, https://www.
   healthline.com/health/mens-health/how-long-does-it-take-for-
   sperm-to-regenerate#sperm-production-rate.

Day 5

1. "How Your Lungs Get the Job Done," American Lung Association,
   July 20, 2017, https://www.lung.org/blog/how-your-lungs-work.

Day 6

1. Robby Berman, "Having a Senses of Purpose May Help You
   Live Longer, Research Shows," Medical News Today, November
   21, 2022, https://www.medicalnewstoday.com/articles/longevity-
   having-a-purpose-may-help-you-live-longer-healthier.
2. Julianne Holt-Lunstad, Timothy B. Smith, and J. Bradley Layton,
   "Social Relationships and Mortality Risk: A Meta-analytic Review,"
   PLoS Medicine 7, no. 7 (July 27, 2010): e1000316, https://journals.
   plos.org/plosmedicine/article?id=10.1371/journal.pmed.1000316.

Day 8

1. Timothy V. Pyrkov et al., "Longitundinal Analysis of Blood
   Markers Reveals Progressive Loss of Resilience and Predicts
   Human Lifespan Limit," *Nature Communications* 12, no. 2765
   (2021), https://www.nature.com/articles/s41467-021-23014-1.

Day 37

1. Charles M. Kilo and Eric B. Larson, "Exploring the Harmful
   Effects of Healthcare," *Journal of the American Medical Association*
   302, no. 1 (2009): 91, https://jamanetwork.com/journals/jama/
   article-abstract/184158.

Day 39

1. Sandra Lopez-Leon et al., "Psychotropic Medication in Children
   and Adolescents in the United States in the Year 2004 vs. 2014,"
   Daru 26, no. 1 (September 2018): 5–10, https://www.ncbi.nlm.nih.
   gov/pmc/articles/PMC6154488/.

2. Adrienne Santos-Longhurst, "Type 2 Diabetes Statistics and Facts," Healthline, updated August 14, 2020, https://www.healthline.com/health/type-2-diabetes/statistics#Age.

3. *2009 Almanac of Chronic Disease* (Partnership to Fight Disease, 2009), 2.

4. Qiuping Gu et al., "Prescription Cholesterol-Lowering Medication Use in Adults Aged 40 and Over: United States, 2003–2012," National Center for Health Statistics Data Brief no. 177, Centers for Disease Control and Prevention, December 2014, https://www.cdc.gov/nchs/products/databriefs/db177.htm.

5. "CDC's Work on Developmental Disabilities," Centers for Disease Control and Prevention, reviewed May 16, 2022, https://www.cdc.gov/ncbddd/developmentaldisabilities/about.html.

6. "Childhood Obesity Facts," Centers for Disease Control and Prevention, reviewed May 17, 2022, https://www.cdc.gov/obesity/data/childhood.html.

7. Debra J. Brody and Qiuping Gu, "Antidepressant Use Among Adults: United States, 2015–2018," National Center for Health Statistics Data Brief no. 377, Centers for Disease Control and Prevention, September 2020, https://www.cdc.gov/nchs/products/databriefs/db377.htm.

8. "Cancer Statistics," National Cancer Institute, updated September 25, 2020, https://www.cancer.gov/about-cancer/understanding/statistics.

9. "Heart Disease Facts," Centers for Disease Control and Prevention, reviewed October 14, 2022, https://www.cdc.gov/heartdisease/facts.htm.

DAY 44

1. Ada McVean, "Broken Bones Grow Back Stronger… Sort Of," McGill Office for Science and Society, April 19, 2018, https://www.mcgill.ca/oss/article/did-you-know/broken-bones-grow-back-stronger-sort.

DAY 45

1. Dean Ornish, MD, "Integrative Care: A Pathway to a Healthier Nation," Senate health reform testimony, Senate Dirksen Building,

February 26, 2009, https://www.help.senate.gov/imo/media/doc/Ornish.pdf.

2. "Heart Disease Rate on the Rise," OSF HealthCare, August 11, 2022, https://newsroom.osfhealthcare.org/heart-disease-rate-on-the-rise/.

DAY 46

1. Justin McCarthy, "Big Pharma Sinks to the Bottom of U.S. Industry Rankings," Gallup, September 3, 2019, https://news.gallup.com/poll/266060/big-pharma-sinks-bottom-industry-rankings.aspx.

DAY 48

1. Dietrich Bonhoeffer, *The Cost of Discipleship* (New York: Touchstone, 1995), 43–45.

DAY 49

1. E. Kalon et al., "Psychological and Neurobiological Correlates of Food Addiction," *International Review of Neurobiology* 129 (2016): 85–100, https://doi.org/10.1016/bs.irn.2016.06.003.

DAY 50

1. Amanda Logan, "Can Expressing Gratitude Improve Your Mental, Physical Health?," Mayo Clinic Health System, December 6, 2022, https://www.mayoclinichealthsystem.org/hometown-health/speaking-of-health/can-expressing-gratitude-improve-health.

DAY 51

1. "About the TSCA Chemical Substance Inventory," U.S. Environmental Protection Agency, updated June 29, 2022, https://www.epa.gov/tsca-inventory/about-tsca-chemical-substance-inventory#whatdoesitmean.

2. Cory Gerlach, "New Toxic Substances Control Act: An End to the Wild West for Chemical Safety?," Science in the News Boston, Harvard University, October 25, 2016, https://sitn.hms.harvard.edu/flash/2016/new-toxic-substances-control-act-end-wild-west-chemical-safety/.

3. Rebecca Harrington, "The EPA Has Only Banned These 9 Chemicals—Out of Thousands," *Business Insider*, February 10, 2016, https://www.businessinsider.com/epa-only-restricts-9-chemicals-2016-2.

DAY 60

1. Penelope Bryant et al., "Antibiotics Before Birth and in Early Life Can Affect Long-Term Health," The Conversation, June 28, 2018, https://theconversation.com/antibiotics-before-birth-and-in-early-life-can-affect-long-term-health-97778.

DAY 61

1. Desonta Holder, "Health: Beware Negative Self-Fulfilling Prophecy," *Seattle Times*, January 2, 2008, https://www.seattletimes.com/seattle-news/health/health-beware-negative-self-fulfilling-prophecy/; "Can Just Telling a Man He Has Cancer Kill Him?," Channel 4 News, November 14, 2011, https://www.channel4.com/news/can-just-telling-a-man-he-has-cancer-kill-him.

DAY 63

1. Wayne Drash, "Not Exercising Worse for Your Health than Smoking, Diabetes, and Heart Disease, Study Reveals," CNN Health, updated January 11, 2019, https://www.cnn.com/2018/10/19/health/study-not-exercising-worse-than-smoking/index.html.

DAY 64

1. Cecily Heslett, Sherri Hedberg and Haley Rumble, "Did You Ever Wonder What's in…?" (student project, Breastfeeding Course for Health Care Providers, Douglas College, New Westminster, BC, Canada, 2007), https://forms.lamaze.org/WhatsinBreastmilkPoster.pdf.

DAY 69

1. See, for instance, "Evidence-Based Lifestyle Protocols, Wellness and Prevention," accessed February 17, 2023, https://www.wellnessandprevention.com/common/printinfo.cfm?id=ABBB8C63-248C-C01C-3E7149224C070827.

DAY 73

1. Gael McGill, "Cellular Landscape," accessed February 17, 2023, https://gaelmcgill.artstation.com/projects/Pm0JL1.

DAY 74

1. Stephanie Cold, "Pottenger's Cats: Early Epigenetics and Implications for Your Health," Price–Pottenger, November 13,

2014, https://price-pottenger.org/blog/pottengers-cats-early-epigenetics-and-implications-for-your-health/.

DAY 76

1. Mary Kekatos, "Viral Photo of a Mother's Milk Proves Why Breast *Is* Always Best," *Daily Mail* (UK), February 10, 2017, https://www.dailymail.co.uk/health/article-4213320/Viral-photo-mother-s-milk-proves-breast-best.html.

DAY 80

1. Bill Gaultiere, PhD, "Fear Not…365 Days a Year," CBN, October 21, 2011, https://www1.cbn.com/soultransformation/archive/2011/10/21/fear-not.-365-days-a-year.

DAY 105

1. Charles Q. Choi, "Humans Glow in Visible Light," NBC News, July 22, 2009, https://www.nbcnews.com/id/wbna32090918.

DAY 109

1. Ashley Hamer, "How Many Megapixels Is the Human Eye?," Discovery, August 1, 2019, https://www.discovery.com/science/mexapixels-in-human-eye.

DAY 122

1. David Mikkelson, "Thomas Edison on the 'Doctor of the Future,'" Snopes, April 17, 2006, https://www.snopes.com/fact-check/the-doctor-of-the-future/.

DAY 131

1. John Staughton, "The Human Brain vs. Supercomputers…Which One Wins?," Science ABC, updated January 17, 2022, https://www.scienceabc.com/humans/the-human-brain-vs-supercomputers-which-one-wins.html.

DAY 133

1. "Body Burden: The Pollution in Newborns," Environmental Working Group, July 14, 2005, https://www.ewg.org/research/body-burden-pollution-newborns; Tom Perkins, "'Forever Chemicals' Found in All Umbilical Cord Blood in 40 Studies," *The Guardian* (US edition), September 23, 2022, https://www.theguardian.com/environment/2022/sep/23/forever-chemicals-found-umbilical-cord-blood-samples-studies.

Day 138

1. Walter C. Willet, "Balancing Life-Style and Genomics Research for Disease Prevention. (Viewpoint)," *Science* 296, no. 5568 (2002): 695, *Gale OneFile: Health and Medicine*, accessed January 31, 2023, https://go.gale.com/ps/i.do?id=GALE%7CA86062235&sid=google Scholar&v=2.1&it=r&linkaccess=abs&issn=00368075&p=HRCA &sw=w&userGroupName=anon%7E6973c7bf.

Day 140

1. Martin A. Makary and Michael Daniel, "Medical Error—the Third Leading Cause of Death in the US," *British Medical Journal* (May 3, 2016): 353, https://www.bmj.com/content/353/bmj.i2139.full.

Day 141

1. Robert N. Butler, MD, "Public Interest Report No. 23: Exercise, the Neglected Therapy," *International Journal of Aging and Human Development* 8, no. 2 (1977–78), https://doi.org/10.2190/AM1W-RABB-4PJY-P1PK.

Day 153

1. "Prescription Drugs: Spending, Use, and Prices," Congressional Budget Office, January 2022, https://www.cbo.gov/system/files/2022-01/57050-Rx-Spending.pdf.

Day 162

1. Lance Broy, MD, "Lifestyle Is the Best Medicine," Holzer Family Medicine, accessed February 20, 2023, https://www.holzer.org/preventive-care/lifestyle/.

Day 173

1. "The Influencer Report: Engaging Gen Z and Millennials," Morning Consult, 2019, https://morningconsult.com/wp-content/uploads/2019/11/The-Influencer-Report-Engaging-Gen-Z-and-Millennials.pdf.

Day 175

1. Kari Oakes, "U.S. Life Expectancy Down; Drug Overdose, Suicide Up Sharply," CenterPointe Hospital, May 27, 2022, https://www.centerpointehospital.com/about/blog/u-s-life-expectancy-down-drug-overdose-suicide-up-sharply/.

DESIGNED TO HEAL

Day 178

1. Christa Sgobba, "Here's When You're Most and Least Likely to Have a Heart Attack," *Men's Health*, July 11, 2017, https://www.menshealth.com/health/a19524979/heart-attack-timing/.

Day 188

1. JAMA and Archives Journals, "Height Loss in Older Men Associated with Increased Risk of Heart Disease, Death," Science Daily, December 12, 2006, https://www.sciencedaily.com/releases/2006/12/061212091850.htm.

Day 194

1. William Mayle, "One Workout Trick That's Proven to Double Your Fat Burn, Says Study," Eat This, Not That, March 17, 2021, https://www.eatthis.com/news-fasted-cardio/.

Day 196

1. KiKi Bochi, "Exercise Linked to Lower Risk for 13 Types of Cancer," Baptist Health, June 7, 2016, https://baptisthealth.net/baptist-health-news/exercise-linked-lower-risk-13-types-cancer.

Day 208

1. Barry Popik, "Truth Sounds Like Hate to Those Who Hate the Truth," Friday, February 28, 2020, https://www.barrypopik.com/index.php/new_york_city/entry/truth_sounds_like_hate.

Day 209

1. David Pride, "Viruses Can Help Us as Well as Harm Us," *Scientific American*, December 1, 2020, https://www.scientificamerican.com/article/viruses-can-help-us-as-well-as-harm-us/.

2. "If the Germ Theory of Disease Were Correct, There'd Be No One Living to Believe It," Howie Chiropractic, June 1, 2018, https://howiechiropractic.com/blog/49971-if-the-germ-theory-of-disease-were-correct-thered-be-no-one-living-to-believe-it.

Day 212

1. Reena Mukamal, "How Humans See in Color," American Academy of Ophthalmology, June 8, 2017, https://www.aao.org/eye-health/tips-prevention/how-humans-see-in-color.

Day 214

1. "Exercise for Your Health," Spine and Health, May 24, 2012, https://www.spineandhealth.com.au/exercise-health/.

Day 215

1. Mercey Livingston, "Doctors Warn That Sugar Can Temporarily Weaken Your Immune System," CNET, June 9, 2020, https://www.cnet.com/health/nutrition/sugar-can-lower-your-immune-system/.

Day 221

1. Chrysoula Boutari and Christos S. Mantzoros, "A 2022 Update on the Epidemiology of Obesity and a Call to Action: As Its Twin COVID-19 Pandemic Appears to Be Receding, the Obesity and Dysmetabolism Pandemic Continues to Rage On," *Metabolism* 133 (August 2022): 155217, https://doi.org/10.1016/j.metabol.2022.155217.

Day 235

1. "Church and Religious Charitable Giving Statistics," Nonprofits Source, accessed February 20, 2023, https://nonprofitssource.com/online-giving-statistics/church-giving/.

Day 242

1. Bhanvi Satija, "U.S. Experts Recommend Weight-Loss Drugs for Obese Children," Reuters, January 9, 2023, https://www.reuters.com/world/us/us-experts-recommend-weight-loss-drugs-obese-children-2023-01-09/.

Day 261

1. Chart used with permission of Dr. Irving Kirsch, author of *The Emperor's New Drugs* (New York: Basic Books, 2011).
2. Liye Zou et al., "Effects of Mind-Body Exercises (Tai Chi/Yoga) on Heart Rate Variability Parameters and Perceived Stress: A Systematic Review With Meta-Analysis of Randomized Controlled Trials," *Journal of Clinical Medicine* 7, no. 11 (October 31, 2018): 404, https://doi.org/10.3390/jcm7110404; Emma Del Carmen Macías-Cortés et al., "Individualized Homeopathic Treatment and Fluoxetine for Moderate to Severe Depression in Peri- and Postmenopausal Women (HOMDEP-MENOP Study): A Randomized, Double-Dummy, Double-Blind, Placebo-Controlled Trial," *PLOS One* 10, no. 3 (March 13, 2015): e0118440, https://

doi.org/10.1371/journal.pone.0118440; "Macías-Cortés 2015," Homeopathy Research Institute, accessed February 28, 2023, https://www.hri-research.org/resources/homeopathy-the-debate/macias-cortes-2015/; Arif Khan et al., "A Systematic Review of Comparative Efficacy of Treatments and Controls for Depression," *PLOS One* 7, no. 7 (July 30, 2012): e41778, https://doi.org/10.1371/journal.pone.0041778.

3. "No Evidence That Depression Is Caused by Low Serotonin Levels, Finds Comprehensive Review," University College London News, July 20, 2022, https://www.ucl.ac.uk/news/2022/jul/no-evidence-depression-caused-low-serotonin-levels-finds-comprehensive-review.

DAY 307

1. James Gallagher, "Fasting Diet 'Regenerates Diabetic Pancreas,'" BBC News, February 24, 2017, https://www.bbc.com/news/health-39070183.

DAY 310

1. Karen Kangas Dwyer and Marlina M. Davidson, "Is Public Speaking Really More Feared Than Death?," *Communication Research Reports* 29, no. 2 (April 30, 2012): 99–107, https://doi.org/10.1080/08824096.2012.667772.

DAY 319

1. Jacqueline Howard, "US Spends Most on Health Care but Has Worst Health Outcomes among High-Income Countries, New Report Finds," CNN Health, January 31, 2023, https://www.cnn.com/2023/01/31/health/us-health-care-spending-global-perspective/index.html.

DAY 325

1. Dr. Josh Axe, "Omega-3 Fatty Acids: Benefits for the Heart, Brain, Joints and More," Dr. Axe, October 26, 2022, https://draxe.com/nutrition/omega-3-fatty-acids/; Leslie Stanton, "How Omega-3 Fights Depression," *Life Extension*, May 2022, accessed February 20, 2023, https://www.lifeextension.com/magazine/2016/7/how-omega-3-fights-depression?gclid=EAIaIQobChMI_JPTvqyf_QIVRsSGCh0g7gD0EAAYBCAAEgIyqvD_BwE.

DAY 341

1. "Mother Teresa Quotes," AZ Quotes, accessed February 28, 2023, https://www.azquotes.com/quote/809106.

DAY 344

1. Robert L. Leahy, "How Big a Problem Is Anxiety?," *Psychology Today*, April 30, 2008, https://www.psychologytoday.com/us/blog/anxiety-files/200804/how-big-problem-is-anxiety.

DAY 346

1. Eric Schlosser and Charles Wilson, *Chew On This: Everything You Don't Want to Know about Fast Food* (New York: Penguin, 2006), 85–86, https://archive.org/details/chewonthis0000schl/page/n5/mode/2up.

DAY 350

1. Christina D. Bethell et al., "A National and State Profile of Leading Health Problems and Health Care Quality for US Children: Key Insurance Disparities and Across-State Variations," *Academic Pediatrics* 11, no. 3 (May–June 2011): S22–S33, https://pubmed.ncbi.nlm.nih.gov/21570014/.

2. Paul W. Newacheck and William R. Taylor, "Childhood Chronic Illness: Prevalence, Severity, and Impact," *American Journal of Public Health* 82, no. 3 (March 1992): 364–71, https://jamanetwork.com/journals/jamapediatrics/article-abstract/515952.

3. Child Neurology Foundation, accessed February 17, 2023, https://www.childneurologyfoundation.org/.

4. "Generation 'Could Die Before Their Parents' as Avoidable Health Complaints Soar," *Daily Mail* (UK), April 13, 2010, https://www.dailymail.co.uk/health/article-1265600/Generation-die-parents-avoidable-health-complaints-soar.html.

DAY 352

1. "Can Upper Cervical Help Me?" Shift Health Center, accessed February 20, 2023, https://www.theshifttc.com/can-upper-cervical-help-me/.

DAY 362

1. "Daily Aspirin Therapy: Understand the Benefits and Risks," Mayo Clinic, October 15, 2021, https://www.mayoclinic.org/

diseases-conditions/heart-disease/in-depth/daily-aspirin-therapy/
art-20046797.

Day 363

1. Clay Wireston, "Jeb Bush Says Americans Consume Vast Majority of Addictive Painkillers," PolitiFact, February 4, 2016, https://www.politifact.com/factchecks/2016/feb/04/jeb-bush/jeb-bush-says-americans-consume-vast-majority-addi/#:~:text=And%20Bush's%20larger%20point%20that,percent%20of%20the%20world%20population.

ABOUT THE AUTHOR

Ben Rall, DC, was born and raised in the Great Plains of South Dakota. There he owned and operated one of the largest chiropractic and wellness clinics in the United States. Currently he is the owner and operator of Achieve Wellness, a chiropractic and wellness clinic that helps individuals, businesses, and churches apply a vitalistic model of health care to their lives. He is also the founder and cohost of the highly rated *Designed to Heal* podcast. For the past twenty years Dr. Rall has passionately served tens of thousands of patients, helping them discover they were designed to heal by our Creator. He lives with his wife, Megan, and two children, Grace and Jack, in Orlando, Florida.

ACHIEVE
WELLNESS

For more information, visit Achievewellness.clinic or scan the QR codes. For speaking and prayer requests, email him at Benrall@mac.com.

Instagram:
@achievewellnessclinic

Instagram:
@designedtohealpodcast

Designed to Heal podcast